D0523375

The

Nurse

as

Healer

Delmar Publishers' Online Services

To access Delmar on the World Wide Web, point your browser to:

http://www.delmar.com/delmar.html

To access through Gopher: gopher://gopher.delmar.com

(Delmar Online is part of "thomson.com", an Internet site with information on
more than 30 publishers of the International Thomson Publishing organization.)

For information on our products and services:

email: info@delmar.com

or call 800-347-7707

The

Nurse

as

Healer

Lynn Keegan, PhD, RN

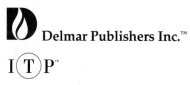

Delmar Publishers Inc.™

I T P™

NOTICE TO THE READER

Cover Design: J² Designs

Delmar staff:
Publisher: David C. Gordon
Senior Acquisitions Editor: Bill Burgower
Assistant Editor: Debra M. Flis
Project Editor: Danya M. Plotsky
Production Coordinator: Barbara A. Bullock
Art and Design Coordinators: Megan K. Desantis
　　　　　　　　　　　　　　Timothy J. Conners

For information, address

Delmar Publishers Inc.
3 Columbia Circle, Box 15015,
Albany, NY 12212-5015

Printed in the United States of America
Published simultaneously in Canada
by Nelson Canada,
a division of The Thomson Corporation

　2 3 4 5 6 7 8 9 10 XXX 00 99 98 97 96

Library of Congress Cataloging-in-Publication Data

Keegan, Lynn.
　　The nurse as healer / Lynn Keegan.
　　　　p. cm. — (Real nursing series)
　　Includes index.
　　ISBN 0-8273-6156-4
　　1. Nursing—Psychological aspects. 2. Healing—Psychological aspects. 3. Nurse and patient. I. Title.
II. Series.
　　[DNLM: 1. Philosophy, Nursing. 2. Nursing Care. WY 100 K26n 1993]
RT86.K44 1993
610.73—dc20
DNLM/DLC

93-26361
CIP

RealNursing Series
Alice M. Stein, MA, RN, Series Editor
Medical College of Pennsylvania

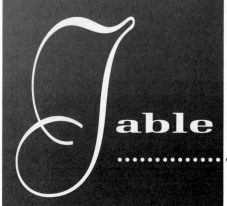

Table of Contents

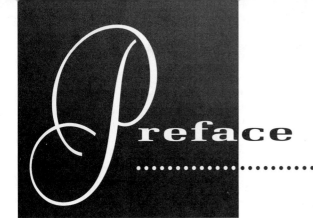

Preface

How do nurses become healers? Are they born that way or can this trait be learned? When studying the myths and legends of healers of the past, it almost seems as if some were born with magical qualities. Yet in my several decades of observation in the healing professions I have encountered many nurses with seemingly gifted healing personalities. Throughout the years I have come to believe that healing attitudes and behaviors are not traits with which only a few chosen are born, but rather that healing is an art and skill that can be learned, developed, and nurtured.

When I was an undergraduate at Cornell University—New York Hospital School of Nursing, I was invited to participate in a senior honors class seminar on healing.

Throughout the following year our small group was uniquely guided through a process designed to enhance the healing qualities we had demonstrated during the selection process. In small intimate classes we met with famous healing greats. Margaret Mead, Rene Dubois, and others came and sat around a table to speak with us, not so much about their theories but about their personal lives and creative thought processes. There within the ivory towers in the heart of New York City, the question was considered: What are healing qualities, and how can they be fostered? Four of us had been chosen because of preexisting attitudes and behaviors that this book discusses: compassion, intent, discipline, listening, and caring. It is my belief that these attitudes and behaviors, once identified, can be nurtured and developed to mold any motivated nurse into an effective healer.

Many contemporary academicians and practicing nurses struggle to find the balance between art and science. We question how much emphasis should be given to the sciences such as pathophysiology, statistics and research. In a packed curriculum how can we teach and integrate the arts? How does the art of nursing relate to desired outcomes? The answers lie in part in the outcome we hope to achieve.

Do we want to become nurse generalists, nurse scientists, nurse practitioners, and is it important to develop a cadre of nurse healers? Is it possible that one nurse can possess multiple qualities?

It is my belief that most people are born with the potential to be healers. To become a truly effective nurse it is important to both build a scientific base and develop healing qualities. I believe that the qualities that are explored in this text on nurse healers are essential to the full development of all nurses.

Special thanks to my editor William Burgower for breathing life into this project.

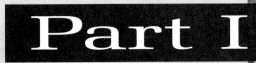

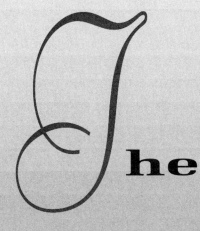

Part I

The Nature of Healing

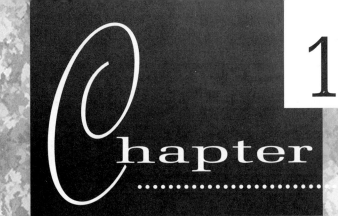

Chapter 1

The Nature of Healing

HEALING

The root of the word "heal" is derived from the Middle English word, "hal", meaning to make whole. Healing, therefore, can be defined as the integration of the totality of humankind in body, mind, and spirit. The healer, then, is one who is capable of producing or catalyzing that integration.

The tradition of healing is far older than the profession of nursing; therefore, it behooves us to explore some of the various theories regarding the nature of healing. Primitive people who had no scientific knowledge knew intuitively that healing was to make whole. Today research shows that their intuitive sense was correct. Their attitudes and behaviors served, then as now, as the basis for healing.

Healing occurs in a variety of ways. Some believe it is primarily spiritual, while others reject the notion of spirituality, believing physiological or physical cures are the only healing possible. The actual mechanism of healing is still unknown. Several categories of healing are described here, showing a variety of currently accepted theories.

TYPES OF HEALING

Faith Healing

Based on prayer and religious faith, healing within this domain occurs because the faith of the supplicant has been answered by the mysterious power of the divine. Cures such as the ones at Lourdes and other holy shrines fall within this category. The method of prayer is common to evangelical practitioners, charismatics, and some one-on-one relationship counselors.

Mind Cures

Healing in this domain relates to the supposition that the diseased states of the body are caused by an aberrant or confused condition of the mind. Adherents to this method attempt to change the state of the mental processes of the client or patient, hence the development of the term "mental therapies." Many contemporary practitioners and groups engage in mind cures. Psychiatric nurses and holistic practitioners subscribe to this belief system to some extent. Groups such as Scientology, Concept Therapy, Humanetics, Silva Mind Control, and others use some portion of this thesis in their healing work.

Metaphysical or Mental Healing

Healers following Christian Science and related systems believe in the nonreality of matter. They assume that our bodies are not real and that, consequently, there is no such thing as disease. They feel that the manifestation of illness and disease is solely an aberration of the mind. Other esoteric metaphysical groups also subscribe to this conceptual belief.

Spiritualism

Historically this system was derived from the belief that spirits of the dead could operate directly, or indirectly through a medium, to heal a patient. In recent years spiritualism has evolved the belief that the source of healing is directed from the Holy Spirit or some greater source flowing into and through the physical form. It is unclear if the healing occurs from the realignment of the molecular structure or from an infusion of light into the cellular substance.

Mesmerism

This system was founded on the supposition that in each person there exists a vital fluid, the free circulation of which results in a state of health and the blocking of the effects of disease. It was believed that this vital fluid could be transmitted to another at will if the recipient was willing to receive and that the movement of the fluid in the recipient provided therapeutic action.

Energy Medicine and Aura Fields

This theory has grown in popularity during the past decade deriving part of its origin from mesmerism and the esoteric practices that were popular during the 1800s. This practice has also been augmented and intertwined with the belief in Oriental meridian theories and the Indian science of chakras. Energy and aura theory is based on the belief that energy fields surround the physical body. These fields can be altered by a practitioner moving the energy through the aural field that surrounds the patient's body. The purpose of the practice is to open blocked channels and, thereby, realign the unbalanced energy system. An entire school of practice has developed based on this theory. Therapeutic touch, aura healing, chakra opening or closing, and electromagnetic healings all fall within this domain.

Hypnotism

In this method it is believed that persons in the hypnotic condition can be controlled by the power of suggestion. Suggestion can be used by the hypnotists to control pain, alter body functions, and change life-style habits. This has become a popular method for smoking cessation and behavior modification. Subliminal tapes use this technique to subtly direct listeners to change their behaviors.

Germ Theory

The entire field of Western scientific medicine has developed around this theory. Practitioners of this approach believe that all illness and disease are caused by invading pathogenic organisms; that is, bacteria and viruses. Many of these organisms can be prevented from entering the body with simple preventative techniques such as personal hygiene, public sanitation, and inoculations of vaccines. It is common for people to be immunized with smallpox, tetanus, pertussis, diphtheria, polio, measles, and mumps vaccines. When one does become ill, scrupulous measures are then used to prevent the pathogenic organism from multiplying. Sterile technique is employed to protect the patient from further pathogen assault when the internal body undergoes surgery. Antibiotic and other pharmaceutical remedies are employed to combat the invading pathogens.

Holistic Health

This view encompasses many of the above theories. Practitioners within this domain believe in the interrelationship of the body, mind, and spirit in an ever-changing environment. Holistic practioners incorporate life-style patterning with other therapies that include the physical, mental, emotional, and spiritual aspects of intervention and support.

Many of the healing therapies can be performed by an accomplished individual on his or her own behalf. It is more common, however, for another person serving as a conduit or channel to facilitate the process. The inclusion of these theories by a practicing nurse healer does not negate the significance of the curative nature of modern technological medicine. Instead these theories offer alternative explanations of why patients get better in many cases despite, or without the benefit of, modern allopathic medicine.

THE NURSE HEALER

Nurse healers come from all walks of life. No matter what our origins, each of us has the capacity to become a healer when we recognize and acknowledge our feelings, attitudes, and behaviors. These traits are not isolated. Our thoughts, emotions, and reactions are literally translated into body changes. We have the capacity to cause internal physiological changes through mind modulation. Conscious or unconscious mental thoughts can stimulate and affect all the systems of our body: autonomic and central nervous systems and the endocrine, immune, and neuropeptide systems. All body systems are affected by how we think, what we eat, how we behave, and the choices we make. It is when we recognize and acknowledge our body-mind connection that we begin to awaken the healer within.

Self-healing or the healing of others can become blocked in times of stress and crisis. With this in mind, it is important to continually assess who we are and what we are doing as we endeavor not only to heal others but to continually work on healing ourselves. So how do we go about getting in touch with the archetype of the Self? Jung believed this was possible only through the phenomenon of relationships. He believed that the self does not become conscious by itself but through the tradition of knowing and individuation. Individuation is possible only through a relationship with one's environment and through contact with like-minded individuals with whom significant relationships can be established (Jung, 1973).

We evolve as healers when we participate in our own healing processes through relationships and attunement with our environment. As we move farther and farther from the primitive aspects of things and closer to the higher domains, we become more intensively involved in both the healing and the growth processes.

THE NURSE AS GUIDE

A nurse healer uses the art of guiding to help others discover and recognize new health behaviors and discover insights about how to make choices and how to cope effectively. Guiding is a special art and intervention that nurses may use anytime. The purpose of guiding is to bring to the present moment the client's fullest potential. The nurse then uses this process to help clients become congruent with their inner resources, decrease stress, and enhance direction toward balance and harmony (Dossey, 1988).

Characteristics of a Nurse Healer

Dossey lists the characteristics of a nurse healer, which include the following:

- Has the awareness that self-healing is a continual process
- Is familiar with the terrain of self-development
- Recognizes weaknesses and strengths
- Is open to self-discovery
- Continues to develop clarity about life's purpose to keep us from acting mechanical and feeling bored
- Is aware of present and future steps in personal growth
- Models self-care to help self and clients with the inward process
- Is aware that his or her presence is equally as important as technical skills
- Respects and loves clients regardless of who or how they are
- Offers the client methods for working on life issues
- Guides the client in discovering creative options
- Presumes that the client knows the best life choices
- Listens actively
- Empowers clients to recognize that they can cope with life processes
- Shares insights without imposing personal values and beliefs
- Accepts what clients say without judging
- Sees time with clients as being there to listen to and dialogue with them, also to serve and share

Self—Identify as a Nurse Healer

Oliver (1990) asked nurses at a college conference in the Northeast how many considered themselves to be healers. Ninty-four percent , 52 out of 55 participants, answered they did. When further asked to identify the healing behaviors they used, the most commonly cited ten behaviors related to healing others. They were as follows:

1. Touching
2. Listening
3. Praying
4. Caring
5. Laughing
6. Crying
7. Using music

8. Dancing
9. Using colors
10. Holding/hugging

Oliver probed further by doing a literature search of the CINAHL computer data base. The cumulative findings were fourteen articles from 1966 to1989 that discussed the "nurse as healer" or "healing" interventions. All fourteen articles were published in the late 1980s and include the following:

1. Four articles on specific healing modalities: hope, faith, touch, and the human voice
2. One article specific to holistic nursing interventions
3. Two personal accounts of nurses as healers
4. Seven articles on therapeutic touch

Oliver's conclusions were that most nurses are poised on the threshold of identifying themselves and their work as healing.

In the next section you will meet contemporary, practicing nurses who self-identify as nurse healers. They are among the growing cadre of nurses who have added the dimension of conscious healing to their scope of nursing practice.

REFERENCES

Dossey, B., Keegan, L., Guzzetta, C., & Kolkmeier, L. Nurse as healer: Toward the inward journey, *Holistic nursing, a handbook for practice.* Gaithersburg, Md: Aspen Publishers, 1988.

Jung, C. G. *AION.* Princeton: Princeton University Press, 1973.

Oliver, N. Nurse, are you a healer? *Nursing forum*, 1990, *25*(2), 11–14.

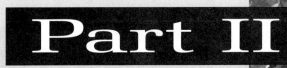

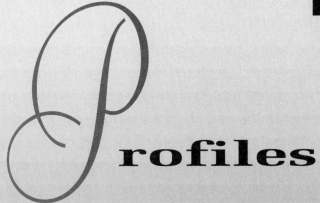

Part II

Profiles

of

Nurse

Healers

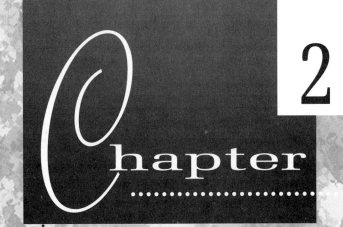

Chapter 2

Profiles of Selected Nurse Healers

Throughout this book there are anecdotal examples of nurse healers. But who are they really? When you read the abstract written word, you use your imagination to conjure up images of who the healers are. In real life, however, they may be different from those in your imagination.

In this chapter you will read about and see real, living, practicing nurse healers. These women and men live and work throughout the world. They write in their own words to describe their personal and professional journies and how they use healing in their nursing practices. They are only a few of the thousands of nurse healers but are representative of nurse healers and of the range of clinical practice they have.

Nurse healers work in every area of nursing:
- Acute care
- Long-term care
- Nursing education
- Consultation and literature
- Entrepreneurs in private practice
- Mental health
- Hospice and home health

Do you view yourself as a nurse healer? Perhaps as you read these stories and see these healers, you will find one, two, or more with whom you can identify. Perhaps then you will respond, yes, I too am a nurse healer.

$\mathcal{L}$inda Smith, MS, RN,
Hospice Director,
Healing Touch Practitioner,
Kentucky

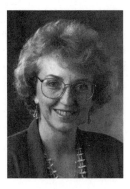

I have often wondered how anyone in an administrative position can be a healer! And yet that is the first description I give to my work now.

A number of years ago I contemplated leaving administration and going back into clinical nursing. I felt I had at some point lost the human side of me that needs to touch and be touched. In dealing with administrative problems and issues, I was becoming "cold-hearted" and it was not a comfortable feeling. Supportive nurse leaders challenged me then to stay in administrative work and help heal nursing. With great timerity I took up that challenge, not knowing how I could help the general situation. Now after years of listening and visioning, I use energy work to heal the healers in my setting—those who care for the dying.

As director of a hospice my overall responsibility is the welfare and care of the terminally ill and their families. I also attend to the staff and volunteers. I have seen stress and what I would call burnout occur when there are not sufficient support systems for all involved. You can well imagine the stress of watching day in, and day out, a loved one deteriorate with no hope of improvement in this life. Families and staff alike make the hand-wringing plea, "Isn't there anything that can be done to ease their suffering?" I think what is happening is an accumulation of stress and pain in the energy field. This occurs not only with the patient but also with family members and staff as well. From observing I have learned to listen with an open heart and then to teach, sometimes by example, how to relax, relieve stress, or connect with a higher spiritual energy. I use touch modalities with staff, patients, and their loved ones to clear the energy field. When patients are involved, I show the staff and family members how to work with the patient to decrease pain and anxiety. Staff sometimes need relief from a headache or just from being "scattered". The expressions on their faces say enough—I have given a gift of relief to those in pain and desperation and of calm to the anxious. It is more than just "giving them something to do" when the pain medications are not working or doing something to them when stress has overtaken their lives. Energy work is an interaction between the energy field of the "healer" and the "healee". Both are affected in the work, bringing a sense of peace and relaxation in the chaotic situation.

For me hospice care is deeply spiritual work. You can not bring a caring touch to another human being without touching the Spirit that binds us all. Energy work allows me to awaken in others their own body-mind-spirit connection. The healers are being healed, and nursing is being reclaimed as the art of touch that it has always been.

Marilee Halo Shames, PhD, RN, Nurse Entrepreneur, California

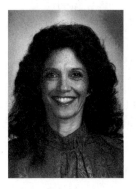

It was in 1976 that I became disillusioned with my job as a psychiatric nurse and with the limitations of Western medicine. My chronic thyroid disorder gave me the opportunity to overcome my fear and work with my body's natural healing potential. It has been my belief that as I delve deeper into my own pain, I become more trustworthy as a "safe container" that others may share deeply with me. My healing journey has been magnificent, teaching me of my personal power and also about the special value of the nurse as health educator, client advocate, and life-transition guide.

Since then I have developed a very holistic approach to healing. I now have a private practice specializing in women's care, which utilizes all the training and education I have ever received. Though grounded in science, my work is intuitive and highly personalized, corresponding to the beliefs and goals of the client. Much of my time is spent in active listening, to ascertain how I can best provide support to empower the clients to meet their own goals.

The initial consultation lasts an hour and a half. During this period I provide an "energetic assessment" by interviewing the person, paying attention to nonverbal clues such as voice inflection, tone, facial expression, body posturing, and anything that informs me of the person's inner life. Often, with the client's permission, I use my hands to find blocks in her energy field or to relieve immediate discomfort. The tools I find most helpful in my work include emotional release, healing touch, homeopathy, flower remedies, crystal healing, massage, and visualization. With selected clients I also use movement to unlock emotions stored in the body.

I ask questions relating to family and love relationships, life experience, spiritual beliefs, expectations, and visions. When any of these topics have significant emotional charge, I encourage the person to share more, to ascertain how she deals with being upset. When appropriate, in subsequent sessions, I demonstrate certain movements for the client to imitate that are very effective at loosening emotions locked in the body's posture.

Often I have found that a single, emotion-releasing session can dramatically affect a woman's sense of efficacy relative to her life's challenges. As she releases emotionally charged experiences in a safe environment, she can more readily move on in her life, reframing the experience from a less distressed viewpoint. I also deeply respect a person's need to reveal information in her own time frame.

Through the years I have become highly attuned to the many subtle ways in which our energy can become drained through defense mechanisms such as blame, projection, denial, repression, or addictions, however minor and insidious. I gently explore with each client the ways she learned to respond to life's challenges. Together we devise short- and long-term goals to provide more enjoyment and harmony in her life.

I am also blessed to be married to a holistic physician and our clients benefit greatly from the collaborative practice. We have found that there is something deeply nurturing about providing a model of male/female (doctor/nurse) working together and complementing each other's contributions. Sometimes I see the client only once, to add my nursing evaluation to his medical assessment. Often I see the client for a few more sessions or on an ongoing basis if mutually desired. As trust builds, the client's are able to go deeper into their wounding, finding their own pathway to recovery with our support and informed guidance.

Most recently I have acquired a beautiful and calmly nurturing office suite, the new home of Nurse Empowerment Workshops & Services (my motivational seminars and retreats) and my private practice, where I specialize in nurse-counseling. From this healing environment I also market my new book (The Nightingale Conspiracy: Nursing Comes to Power in the 21st Century). My ultimate goal is to inspire nurses to acknowledge and honor themselves for their own special healing gifts. Thus they become increasingly more able to find fulfillment, both personally and professionally. As we heal ourselves, we heal our profession and our world.

Virginia Willis, MS, RN, Director, School of Nursing, Texas

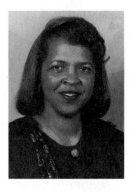

In nursing education, holism is integrated into the curriculum. Educators encourage and engage in studies that add validity to holistic approaches. As educators we view ourselves as nurse healers. We offer ourselves to students. Educators become role models of empowered beings from whom others learn.

In our nursing program holism is well integrated. Not only do we teach about and practice according to holistic concepts, but we also integrate holism into the performance of our jobs.

As a nurse healer I perform a variety of roles to promote growth and life processes that move us toward wholeness. A very important aspect of my role as a nurse healer is using the art of guiding to help faculty and students recognize new paths for fulfilling their potential. Often students come to my office with vague ideas but no real direction. Through the process of helping the student explore possibilities, I am there to point out hazards and precautions, as well as options and potentials.

I also work as a facilitator for students and faculty to assist them in moving in the direction of growth toward wholeness. To accomplish this goal I must listen and share and accept who we are as individuals. In this way, people experience personal empowerment through the encouragement of being coparticipants in the process of educating the student. Nursing students are open to new ideas and are eager to make a difference in the lives of others. Seeds are planted in the educational process.

I am a nurse healer. I see myself as part of the whole, an example of a nurse healer. It is my belief that the concept of holistic nursing does not have to be sold. All we really have to do is just live it ourselves. I want each faculty member and student to see me as an example of one of professionalism, kindness, fairness, and caring. I offer myself. I believe that my being genuine with others makes a difference.

Educators who are fully present in body, mind, and spirit create the healthiest view they can of themselves and of their world. Their very presence makes a difference to students, other colleagues, and society at large.

Lynne Herdrich, MS, FNP, RN, Family Nurse Practitioner, Virginia

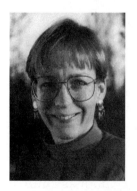

When I became a nurse, I became a nurse practitioner. For the past twelve years I have cared for women in the primary care setting, most recently in a private OB/GYN practice with three nurse practitioners and three physicians. To function as a nurse practitioner I depend on physician comanagement for part of my practice. I would not be prescribing or doing certain procedures without their collaboration. However, much of what I do or say with my clients is nurse/holistic oriented. As I become more experienced in holism/wellness, I downplay the medical model in my practice. Now I am completing my nurse-midwifery studies, moving farther from a physician-oriented setting.

Many of women's health problems stem from the stress of trying to "do it all" with full-time work, marriage, and parenting. Many women lose touch with their bodies, their natural cycles. Nourishment, whether whole foods, emotional support, or meditation is lacking in many women's lives. As I see my clients and counsel them regarding PMS, dysmenorrhea, infertility, or menopause, I work to guide them back to themselves. I ask them to find time to honor what is strong and female about themselves. Always, when I touch or examine a client, I do it from my center with the intent to contact the personal healer within each client. She may also need medication or a referral to a specialist, but it is always my intent to help her find her personal path to wellness. This approach fosters self-responsibility, and that is where real change can take place.

For me to function as a holistic practitioner I must model wellness myself, not only to my clients but to the staff and physicians with whom I work. Usually I am the one who brings in the snacks from the health food store or steamed vegetables from the cafeteria lunch line. They kid me quite a bit about being the health nut, but they notice. Also they notice when I "regress" and have a cup of coffee or grab a Twinkie. So we talk about why we eat what we do and how old habits reemerge. My hope is that as the staff become models for wellness, the whole office will function in wellness. Then our clients will begin to notice.

So healing involves really noticing that one is part of the whole picture. This reflects how I care for my clients. As I strive to live in balance, I can begin to touch that personal healer in my clients and we can then make the journey to wellness together.

Dorothea Hover, EdD, RN, Nurse Psychotherapist, California

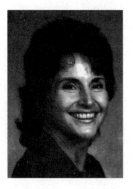

With an extensive background in public health nursing and fifteen years of practice as a licensed psychotherapist, I have arrived at a new integration by developing the concept of myself as a nurse healer. Practicing both as a nurse and as a psychotherapist, I offer energy-based healing work through my private practice in San Diego. Oftn by the time clients see me, they have exhausted all medical resources and simply seek relaxation and pain relief.

For example, a women asked me to visit her dying mother and to help with the transition. I went to the home where hospice nurses were in attendance and found an emaciated sixty-year-old suffering from the terminal stages of AIDS. She found such relief as I worked in her energy field to smooth and facilitate balancing. During the visit I was also able to teach the home-care nurses how to make the patient comfortable by smoothing the field surrounding the physical body and gently placing the hands on tender joints and energy centers. Later, the nurses called me to say that their cranky patient had not slept so well in weeks. This alone was significant to me since medication by itself had not touched the pain or anxiety of the patient. Since I heard nothing further, I assumed Mary had passed on, perhaps more peacefully because of our time together. Six weeks later, Mary called to say she had never felt better than at the time of my treatment and asked to see me again. This time she was able to drive to my office and looked splendid. Again, as during the first session, there was a flood of questions and again the wonderful silence of relaxation as I worked in her energy field using a variety of energy and touch techniques. I included some self-help work to maintain her energy level. Therapeutic issues such as resolving old grudges and forgiving her many enemies also came to the surface and could be dealt with at subsequent sessions.

Essentially I am always surprised when things like this happen. I have no expectations of the energy work, or of therapy for that matter, but I do know that the psyche and soma have tremendous capacities for recuperation under the right circumstances. I see my task as making available a healing environment of permission and safety in which the client's innate healing potential can be activated.

Rita Benor, RGN, RM, RHV, NDV, RNT, Cert. Ed.,
Lecturer in Palliative Nursing, London, England

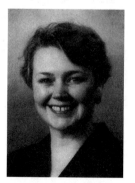

I have witnessed good, easy deaths and difficult deaths, predictable ones and surprising, unexpected ones. With each I have a clear impression or image and still recall the uniqueness of each individual person's transition. It is important to begin to sort out, learn from, and find ways to share our experiences with regard to death. How else will we grow in our abilities to avoid unnecessary suffering and how else will we find ways to teach what we learn?

It is suggested that a good death is one where individuals have had opportunities to be involved in the decisions surrounding their care and disease management; where distressing symptoms and pain are controlled; where support is extended to family or friends; where there is clear communication based on truth and respect of feelings; and where psychological needs are responded to and cared for holistically.

Healing through a holistic framework in terminal illness, even more clearly than in other illnesses, is not about cure but about a gentle, pervasive reaching into all the dimensions of individuals to help them arrive at a state of acceptance. This is not accomplished through passivity but through a gradual awakening or awareness, touching those parts that are damaged, hurting, blocked, or unexpressed. When one develops a quality of wholeness the process of self-healing is initiated.

I work with clients such as "Jim," a 41-year-old married businessman with two small children, who was devastated to learn that he had an advanced cancer in his chest with a life expectancy of 2 to 3 months. Treatment could only be palliative, and he was advised to see the chaplain and to make contact with the local hospice. It was the community hospice nurse who referred him to me for psychotherapy, relaxation, and healing.

During his therapy with me, Jim made great strides in changing his attitude toward death. He became competent and committed to a daily time of relaxation, meditation, and visualization. He read books for inspiration and gradually opened to his feelings. On his final day of life he was helped to his bed and died in peace in the presence of his family.

Years ago as a young nurse of twenty I knew that this part of my awareness about the need for guided transition existed, and yet my professional training had reduced the experience of dying and death to providing comfort. This was tainted with elements of failure because I could not provide cures. As I now work with people who are in the palliative phase of illness and also teach professional nurses, I hope that we may find the ways to ease, explain, explore, and simply allow the natural processes of death transition to take place. This is not only for those who are dying but also for all of those involved in the process. Healing comes in many forms. We must keep our hearts and minds open to the many possibilities and opportunities arising each time we face a transition.

Barbara Dossey, MS, RN, FAAN, Author and Consultant, New Mexico

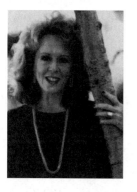

After twenty-eight years of being in the world of health care, the challenge for me with patients, their families, and my colleagues has been to teach rituals that integrate a person's belief systems and their innate healing ability with modern technology. Much of my professional career has been spent with patients and their families as they face cardiovascular disease and critical illness. There have been many technologic breakthroughs in cardiovascular disease such as pacemakers, coronary artery bypass surgery, heart assist devices, and procedures and medications to open up and clean out coronary arteries. However, the causes and cures for many cardiovascular problems still have not been discovered. So we are painfully aware that the sophisticated technology and medications really do not provide all the answers in preventing, stabilizing, and reversing cardiovascular illness. We are also aware that the current Western medical model does not explain the psychological, social, or spiritual causes of the disease. Why then is the medical model still falling short of predicted criteria? Could it be that after all these centuries we now realize that the biomedical model can never provide us with complete answers in treating heart disease, cancer, and other major illnesses? It has never taken into account either the profound devastating effects or the enormous healing effects of a person's mind and spirit on the body. We are at a time in history when we must transform our health care system from a disease management industry to a healing system.

As I have listened to the rich tapestry of patients' life stories, I have realized that the meaning that they gave their lives and the healing rituals that they incorporated for the most part directed how they would heal, almost without regard to medical technology or treatments used. I entered cardiovascular and critical care nursing in the early 1960's at a time when the thoughts, emotions, and beliefs of the patients and families were more valued by physicians and nurses who practiced an authentic kind of healing. As technology increased, so did impersonal interactions, specialization, and a focus on curing of symptoms. When a patient got well, it was attributed to the machines and the potent medications. The meaning of illness and its place and purpose in a person's life became anachronistic.

In the 1970's exciting research on interactions of beliefs and emotions on physiology and healing appeared in leading professional journals. I now had scientific validation of what I had witnessed for over a decade. As I learned more about self-regulation skills and integrated them into my own life, my professional practice also began to change. I began to teach these same self-regulation skills to patients in the critical care unit and in cardiac rehabilitation programs. It was thrilling to participate with patients and their families as they shared their stories and healing rituals with each other and learned how to alter their own biochemistry and decrease their fear and anxiety. For example, patients in significant pain could learn how to distract themselves from the pain with relaxation and imagery exercises; a patient with minimal blood flow to his severely injured left leg used relaxation and imagery skills to increase blood flow to his injured leg and avoided amputation. With a change in attitude and being empowered, these patients' body chemicals and inner healing resources worked toward their recovery rather than to impede their healing. This repeated experience with many patients and their families allowed me to deeply understand the importance of rituals and the rich tapestry of the interconnectedness of body-mind-spirit.

Currently, teaching and writing in the area of self-regulation and healing is my focus. Assisting people to identify their belief systems, their inner world of images, and to find their own pathways to wellness with personal rituals continues to be a healing journey. The joy of facilitating this process deepens my rich experiences as I continue to weave my own caring-healing journey.

Stephen E. Chagnon, RN, Independent Practice, New York

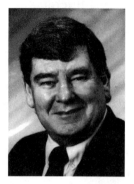

To pursue a vision of service to others, I exchanged a construction engineer's career for a nursing career. This began with a return to school and an A.D.N. from Hahnemann University in 1978. After clinical experiences in rehabilitation, burn units, intensive care units, and agency positions, I was burned out and needed a change. I decided to develop my own practice because people asked for more of my services after regular work hours.

While employed in clinical areas I found my most effective nursing occurred when I provided physical comforts and information about the situation at hand. Today I still do this; only now I am more aware of the holistic nature of the healing process. Today my knowledge is more useful in terms of body function and the range of options for interactions.

I started expanding my nursing skills in 1981 with foot reflexology, body chemistry training, and self-awareness training. Developing new skills has become an endless quest for understanding how the body works and how I can interact with it to get the desired results. This personal-growth path was arduous. I have learned that it is never ending and full of wonderments.

I imagine the body as a pyramid with "thought" at the top, with chemistry below, and with the body below that. Massage assists the body most importantly in wastes and readjusting muscle tension. This process is supported by nutrition (body chemistry), and these together provide the forum for thought, which is the beginning of change to what is wanted.

I first started my independent practice with an office at home. The mortgage quickly created a need to develop marketable skills and to describe them in creditable, understandable ways. Today, 12 years later, my practice is in an office building with a great view of the city and mountains. Here I assist my clients to unravel nature's ways as they develop confidence in their own innate healing process.

Each person I see is unique. Some are trying to improve their bodies' performance by shaving a 0.01 second off their sport's world record. Others come with physical challenges such as muscular dystrophy. Each person is evaluated and then presented with rationales for various massage and body chemistry options from which they create their own treatment plan. Treatment effectiveness is determined by overall body performance and by how well various body functions interact with each other. Using this simple, step-by-step, problem-solving approach, easily replicated by the client, everyone is successful.

I love what I do. The joy I feel inside when a client transforms from a negative, painful stranger to a cheerful, enthusiastic, positive client is greatly rewarding. It is when I help people to help themselves that I feel I am a nurse healer.

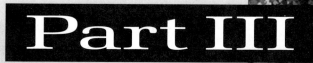

Part III

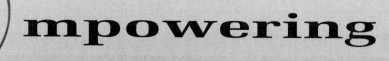

Empowering the Self for Becoming a Healer

Chapter 3

Strengthening the Body-Mind

"So the vital strength of his spirit won through, and he made his way far outside the flaming walls of the world and ranged over the measureless whole, both in mind and spirit."

Lucretius (94–55 B.C.)

Empowering Yourself

What do I like best about myself?

What are my personal strengths?

Do I set and am I able to complete goals I set for myself?

Do I perceive my personal strengths as a way of understanding the patterns of health and illness in my life?

BODY-MIND SYSTEMS

When we recognize that to some extent all of us are wounded and begin to work toward healing our wounds, we are ready to begin strengthening and integrating the body-mind to become whole. This chapter represents a modern extension of the knowledge passed down by countless generations of healers. We are rediscovering the principles of wholeness and interconnectedness of which the shamans, wise women, and classical civilizations told us years ago.

Holism

As our conscious awareness evolves, we begin to understand that we are more than just physical beings; we recognize that we are body, mind, emotion, and spirit beings. The following diagram of the Body-Mind-Spirit Template exemplifies how what we do with any one aspect of our being influences and interrelates with all the other aspects.

FIGURE 3-1
Body-Mind-Spirit Template

	BODY	MIND	SPIRIT
BODY	body body	mind body	spirit body
MIND	body mind	mind mind	spirit mind
SPIRIT	body spirit	mind spirit	spirit spirit

Source: Reprinted from Keegan, L., & Dossey, B. *Self-care: A program to improve your life,* 1987. Used with permission of Bodymind Systems, Temple, Tex.

All of our actions have an effect on our total being. Because of the holistic aspect of our lives, each system has a direct effect on every other system. When we work on one part of our being, all parts change. We are so connected that to change the body is to simultaneously affect the mind and spirit. For example, if you feel stressed and anxious, your body becomes tight and symptoms such as tight muscles and rapid breathing may occur. Once you become aware of these changes, you can mentally induce a deep breathing technique and physically change the effect on your body.

Scientific Foundations for Body-Mind Connections

Psychoneuroimmunology researcher Candace Pert tells us that neuropeptide messenger molecules not only flow through the brain but that the cells themselves may actually "think." Through her work she documents that our mental thought processes manifest in our bodies. Surgeon Bernie Siegel has found that exceptional cancer patients, those who believe they can fight their disease and live, actually do survive longer than their counterparts who give up and give in to their disease. Others are also documenting the body-mind connection. Inherent within this belief in the body-mind connection is the notion that our physical body takes on, holds, and manifests the emotions and thought patterns experienced within our mental and spiritual domains.

All of us undergo dynamic processes that create patterns in our lives. Patterns are always a blend of body, mind, and spiritual expressions of wholeness. We can learn through our conscious ability how to enhance health and decrease the symptoms of disease. The idea of consciousness is central to the continued development and understanding of human potential. When we think in terms of our wholeness, it not only affects attitudes toward others, it also affects our understanding of our connectedness of body, mind, and spirit.

Our own conscious and unconscious mental and emotional reactions and patterning, how we care for our physical being, and the kinds of relationships we choose contribute in some part to the creation of our own illnesses. It is through the conscious realization of and the working on and through these patterns that we have the capacity to strengthen and heal our body-mind. This is not to say that illness or disease is only brought on by our unconscious actions, for this is entirely too limited and discounts the importance of the genetic and germ theories. What is important to acknowledge, however, is that factors other than organisms external to our bodies may play a role in our bodies' functions.

Life Patterns

Human beings are complex feedback loops. As we become aware of these feedback loops, we are able to understand our body-mind connections. Think of all the life experiences that run through your body, mind, and spirit.

Each person has both strengths and weaknesses. Identify your strengths. The time taken to evaluate the source of strengths can help an individual acknowledge a belief system and develop a sense of personal worth. When one says, "My strengths are that I am organized and I learn from my mistakes," these pattern recognitions affect the thought-pattern process. The messages go to the core of one's being. Thoughts connect with our human potentials so that our bodies react with positive responses. When we disclose our strengths, we confirm attitude patterns. Humans must continually search for expressions of their human condition. We have the ability to choose our work, our relationships, and our play to assure that they are reflective of a positive outlook on life.

Health Beliefs

As we begin to care for ourselves, certain health beliefs begin to emerge, which include the following:

- Health is a social, emotional, physical, and spiritual state of being
- Health is a fluid state
- It is possible to learn new health habits
- Illness and stress are related
- As you grow in health, you model the value of good health to others
- Vibrant health is a good investment

Anyone embarking on a path to change or improve their health habits, must begin with self-assessment. Assessment is an important first step to problem-solving and to awareness of where one's strengths and weaknesses lie. Commitment to a program of change begins with the assessment phase, and from the initial assessment comes a sense of self-control which enables the process of change.

Through self-assessment one begins the health-building process. This process consists of awareness of the situation, concern for the process, assessment, and development of the action plan. Any self-care program is an individual matter performed on one's own behalf and done to build and maintain health and well-being.

CIRCLE OF HUMAN POTENTIALS

Life involves many possibilities and potentials. Sometimes these potentials are fully actualized, but more often they are not. The basic human potentials can be represented by a circle, which is an ancient symbol of wholeness. In this model the circle has six separate but equally important parts: physical, mental, emotions, spirit, relationships, and choices. When any part is incomplete, the entire circle loses its strength since all parts create the whole. A handy way to reference and remember the categories is to think of divisions of a pie and consider each piece as an area of human potential.

FIGURE 3-2
Circle of Human Potentials

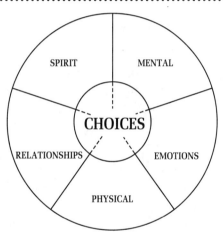

Source: Reprinted from Keegan, L., & Dossey, B. *Self-care: A program to improve your life,* 1987. Used with permission of Bodymind Systems, Temple, Tex.

All of these human potentials are constantly interacting. By becoming aware of our strengths and our weaknesses in each area, we begin to move toward our highest capabilities. When we focus on our whole potential, we begin to understand that real living starts from within and are able to live in accord with our own philosophy of life.

Physical Potential

Everyone's body is unique. The body is a gift to nurture and respect. When the body is nurtured, it increases in strength, vitality, energy, sexuality, and capacity for language and connection with the other potentials. When you strengthen yourself, (1) your own being responds; (2) you actually enhance your general feeling of well-being; and (3) you become a role model with a positive influence on others.

No one gains strength or power without influencing other people in some way. This is especially true of the disabled since they model not only to other disabled but to the nondisabled as well. Consider the role model of Helen Keller who, though she could not see or hear, became an exquisite model of overcoming handicaps. Those with far less disabilities, indeed even those with no physical handicaps at all, looked to her as an example of what is possible for everyone who truly wants to achieve their potential.

As one becomes stronger by eating nutritiously and exercising, he or she becomes healthier and happier. This impacts all the other potentials.

Mental Potential

Our picture of the world is created entirely from mental stimuli. It is through the mind that interest in and knowledge about new life processes occur. When one is open to information, suggestions, and help, mental growth is possible. It is from an open and receptive mental attitude that the healing and creativity unfolds.

In the final stages of T. H. White's *Camelot*, after all has been destroyed and the great King Arthur defeated, Arthur asks the wizard Merlin, What is left? Merlin says, "We can go on learning." The oriental concept "Wei Chi" expresses the same lesson when each mishap is referred to as a teacher. The human brain has unlimited potential if we are willing to tap it. Every experience becomes a part of a lesson. The mind can tap into all sorts of consciousness or by discipline can learn many skills.

Emotional Potential

Emotions are our feelings—our inner and outer responses to the events in our life. One of the greatest challenges we have is to acknowledge, own, express, and understand our emotions. We are living systems constantly interacting with our environment. All life events affect our emotions and general well-being. Some events cause fear. When this occurs, we must not run and hide as if these feelings did not exist. Each of us knows fear just as we know calmness. We must face the fear to understand the meaning. As we become more balanced in living, we allow our humanness to develop. We reach out and ask for human dialogue that is meaningful. Increasing this potential allows our spontaneity and positive, healthy zest for living to emerge. We must be aware of and take responsibility for expressions that allow spirit and intuition to flower.

To maximize this potential we can learn to assess verbal expressions, as well as nonverbal expressions such as voice patterns, posture, gait, general appearance, and facial expressions. Become aware of thought processes. During most of our waking hours we are in constant conversation with ourselves. In fact the person we talk to the most is ourself. What are we reinforcing minute by minute? Our thoughts are literally translated into body changes. If our thoughts are hopeful and optimistic, our body responds with confidence, energy, and hope. On the other hand, if negative thoughts are dominant, our body responds with tightness, uneasiness, and even a change in breathing patterns, blood pressure, and heart rate. Both positive and negative thoughts are daily events.

Emotions are gifts. When we bury them, we lose part of ourselves. There is no such thing as a good or bad emotion. Each is a part of the human condition. These exist as the light and shadow of the self; thus we must acknowledge both of them. They create the dance of life, the polarity of living. We know the light because we know its opposite, the shadow. When we realize the value of both "good" and "bad" emotions, we are then in a position to make effective choices. When we are aware of how body, mind, and spirit are connected, a new sense of making choices for better living can emerge. Focus on acknowledging and understanding all your thoughts for increased health and enthusiasm.

The Role of Emotions In Health

Most of us accept the idea that we "hold" tension in our shoulders or that unrelieved stress can result in a headache. Concurrently, we find that a good massage or some form of relaxation will relieve these somatizations. If we accept these body-mind correlations, then it is not such a big stretch to accept other, more complicated, body-mind relationships. Perhaps the most difficult aspect to face is the idea that our emotions do play a role in our own health or illness. At first it is difficult to look at behavioral patterns in illness. That is because we are only in the frontier of accepting and elucidating which patterns are actually related to which specific illness. However, as more and more of us become aware that there is an emotional/psychological correlation with the health of the biological organism, then we will be on the right track to identifying and matching behavioral patterns with illness and disease.

Many nurses' backgrounds and education have been in the scientific, linear, medical model. From this model we were taught that germs, bacteria, or other external organisms penetrate and invade our bodies and that they make us ill. It is within the limitations of this model that the majority of Western medical practice is based. Traditional practitioners of Western medicine make diagnoses based on the evaluation of a health history, physical examination, and laboratory findings. Treatment follows in the form of pharmaceutical or surgical intervention. Once the symptoms are treated and alleviated, therapy is considered complete. The belief is that organisms invade the body from an external source and that healing transpires through therapy designed to rid the body of the invading pathogen, tumor, or degenerative process either by surgery, antibiotics, or palliative comfort measures. Little or no attention is given to why, at this place and at this time, the pathogen invaded the body in the first place or why the tumor began to grow. It is the exploration of this area of "why here and now" that the new science embraces.

All of us, all the time, are surrounded by potentially pathogenic organisms. They coexist with us in the air that we breathe and on the objects that we touch. For example, we are continually in contact with viruses that cause the common cold. Recent investigations have shown that there are other factors involved in whether we actually develop a cold. Researchers have incubated cold viruses, placed them directly on the mucous lining of the nose, and found that their subjects acquired colds only 6% of the time. The odds were not increased by exposing subjects to cold drafts, putting their feet in water to give them chills, or anything else that was physical. We have begun to learn that there are other, still to be identified, factors, that cause the host to be susceptible to illness, infections, tumor development, or disease.

What about treatment? Most people, when sick, want symptom relief and an antibiotic bacterial assault on the organism producing the symptoms. Therefore, when we develop symptoms, most of us seek medical intervention and use the prescribed pharmaceutical remedies. However, with additional knowledge about our emotional patterning and with increasing awareness of this variable as a possible causative factor, we can play an important part in the healing process. If our emotional suppressions and behavioral patterns are a contributing factor, we need to face and explore this premise and begin to find and utilize ways of effectively dealing with them.

Positive Emotions: Loving Ourselves

If we accept the premise that uncontrolled or negative emotions can contribute to illness and other bodily expressions, what about the effect of positive emotions on our bodies? I believe there is little doubt that when we learn to love and cherish our bodies, they "take on" the internalized love. Most of us have had someone, sometime, who has loved our body. It may have been a lover, or it may have been our mother. Recall how you felt during that loving episode. Most of us respond well and in a healthy manner to the touch and admiration of external love. For the most part, our bodies thrive on it. Rarely are we sickly during the love adventure. If love directed from another creates a state of wellness within, will self-love effectively produce the same result? I believe the answer is yes! If we believe this, then each of us has the capacity to pay attention to and love ourself.

If each of us began the day loving our own bodies through positive affirmations and self-blessing, we would more than likely begin to change patterns within. Ritualized loving attention to our bodies will contribute to their blossoming. When we begin to love ourselves, we pay attention to what we eat, how we exercise, our posture, our appearance, what we think, and how we express ourselves. It is the conscious attention given to loving ourselves that can make the difference in how we feel. When we love ourselves enough, we then have the courage to face our shadows and examine old behavior patterns. With love we have the necessary security to look closely at patterns when things do not go well or when we become ill. Love is the prime ingredient we need to nourish our body-mind and to make us healthy and whole.

Spiritual Potential

The spirit potential is so important that the next entire chapter addresses this domain.

Relationship Potential

We simply cannot live purposeful lives without meaningful relationships. No one lives in isolation. We all have human contacts in different areas—home, work, organizations, and communities. We may not share our home with anyone, but we all live in neighborhoods that are part of communities that make up cities and states. We belong to a nation and, by extension, to the whole planet Earth. Our relationships exist on many different levels ranging from the superficial to the deeply connected.

The challenge in relationships is to extend ourselves and to learn how to exchange our feelings of honesty, trust, intimacy, compassion, openness, and harmony. It is important to share our life process through true interchange with others. Think about how you can increase the dialogue with your family, friends, colleagues at work, and your community at large. It is a skill that requires awareness.

We must identify the harmony, as well as the disharmony, in our relationships. We must identify avenues for change to repattern our life process toward balance and harmony. We must also be aware of the impact we have on our family and friends. We are not isolated. If you are in a good mood, you affect your friends and vice versa. If you are in a bad mood, you also affect your friends. Life is participation. There are no neutral events. Something always occurs when people are together, either positively or negatively. By our attitude and orientation we can affect the outcome of all our encounters.

Right Relationships

To become a truly effective nurse healer you will want to develop consciousness about your relationships. However, development of consciousness is not possible without significant emotional interaction with others. If we have not loved and hated, been inspired and injured by others, then life has not been lived. For this reason relationships are instrumental in our development as healers. However, not just any relationship is enough. For the relationship to be valuable, it must be the kind that makes us vulnerable to scrutinizing ourselves and to being hurt. This means that the decision to become a healer requires risk. We must risk, however, to become whole, and wholeness is an attribute of a healer. It is in the right relationships that we not only succeed but also fail, and when we fail, we learn from our mistakes. However, we are our mistakes, as well as our successes, and that is part of the wholeness. A life without mistakes is impoverished, but growth is the outcome of our increasing consciousness learned through the pain of encountering our shadow.

It is by and large the love relationship that offers the best opportunity for growth. However, we must be careful to differentiate being in love with someone from loving someone. To be "in love" means that a part of oneself is projected onto the other and what you are seeing is your own projected soul image. The danger in this relationship is that you are in fact only loving the projection of yourself. There is an unconscious identification with the other person. The problem occurs when, in time, the humanness of the other begins to become apparent and the magical nature begins to disappear. If based on fantasy and projection, the bond will break and "love" recedes.

If, however, you remain in possession of your own self when you "love someone," you can perceive the other person as they actually are and can commit to care for this person in all their humanness. When you love someone you are mutually affected by each other on an emotional level. When we love and do not run away from the inevitable conflicts, we can be wounded, healed, angered, or enriched. We experience the match of opposites in these close relationships because love and hate, joy and anger are mixed together. Without a doubt loving someone will bring us suffering and personal conflict, but from that the turmoil of soul consciousness and thus wholeness develops. We need right relationships to help us grow from helpers into healers.

Choice Potential

People have an enormous capacity for making choices for their lives. These choices can be conscious or unconscious. Health and balance occur when the skill of effective choice making is utilized. This includes discipline, persistence, goal setting, priorities, action steps, and knowing our options. There is no one way to accomplish any one thing. At all times we must be open to new knowledge and new skills for living. It is when we become active participants in daily living, not passive recipients, that life is good to us.

Each of us is responsible for assessing our own values and desires. No one else can make decisions for us. When we do not exercise our ability to make choices, the beliefs and values of others are imposed on us and we never reach our highest potential.

Making choices involves taking risks. We may make some mistakes along the way, but we also gain experience. Choice involves taking a stand on issues. If we do not take a stand, our ambivalence will keep us stuck. When one continues to develop clarity in life, there is a follow-through on goals.

Summary

Each area of our human potential affects the whole. If one area is undeveloped, one feels that things are not as good as they could be. However, when all areas are developed, a sense of wholeness emerges. One's self-esteem increases and life goals are actualized. Being alive becomes exciting. Even when there are frustrations, the healthy, integrated person is able to recognize choices and move through the blocks.

Healer Reflections

- **What is my belief concerning the relationship of health with stress?**
- **Is there an integration of attention to the body, the mind, and the spirit in my life?**
- **Do I believe that I can work on self-development at the same time that I work to assist others?**
- **Do I have the right relationships in my life to foster the growth process?**

Chapter 4

Discovering the Light Within

"No man, when he hath lighted a candle, putteth it in a secret place, neither under a bushel, but on a candlestick, that they which come in may see the light."

St. Luke

Empowering Yourself

Note that the spiritual journey is an effective means of developing the light within.

Consider the aspects of change that awaken us to the desire for the spiritual journey.

Learn the purpose of the journey and the techniques for fostering the process.

Understand why it is important to be aware that there are factors that inhibit the process.

OUR INNER NATURE

If our deepest inner nature is spiritual, we must be in contact with it to be healers. From the earliest time of the shaman we have witnessed the mysterious spiritual element of healing. Dreams, trances, and altered states of consciousness with the shamans, dream therapy in ancient Greece, and the connection of the healer with the divine have all been part of our evolutionary path.

SPIRITUAL JOURNEYING

Spiritual journeying is a process of unfoldment, a journey of discovering the light within. It is ongoing and continuous and is a part of the life of every healer. The deeper one journeys, the greater the discoveries.

Spirit

Spirituality is a broad concept that encompasses values, meaning, and purpose. The term spirit is derived from several ethnic and historical sources. In Latin it meant "breath." Greeks evolved the term from the root word "wind." Later biblical sources describe spirit as the breath of divinity flowing through us. Buddhists think of spirit in terms of inner light or truth. In contemporary times we have come to think of spirit as divine animation, inner guidance, a higher power, the basic indwelling principle, and in a variety of other conceptual ways.

Webster defines spirit as the breath of life. I believe spirit comprises an entire multitude of animations that are present at every level of existence from the simplest material level to the level of the divine. Perhaps spirit is that which makes the electrons spin around their nucleus and that which affects "animate and inanimate life" within matter. In human beings spirit is elevated to a higher plane and contains not only the animating principle of the lower forms of matter and life but also incorporates the principle of the divine, which many call the soul (the divine spirit within).

The most important thing in defining spirit is the recognition that it is an essential need of human nature. There is something in all of us that seeks the spiritual. This yearning varies in strength from person to person but is always there in everyone. Spirit is experienced when one turns inward to explore the human capacities of honesty, love, caring, wisdom, imagination, and compassion. It is the conscious seeking of the Light, of the Truth, or of the connection with Source that is the beginning point of the spiritual journey.

The Spiritual Journey

Lao Tzu, an ancient Chinese philosopher said, "The journey of a thousand miles must begin with a single step." The personal spiritual journey begins the same way, one step at a time.

The spiritual journey involves the process an individual undergoes in search of the meaning and purpose of life. The journey itself may be literal or figurative, but it entails the spiritual quest of seeking answers to the meaning of life and death.

Historical examples of this phenomenon are found within the rich heritage of the past. There were some individuals, now recognized as saints, who in the midst of traditional religion heard the voice, saw the light, or followed the inward call to a personal spiritual journey. To mention only a few, there were people such as St. Francis of Assisi, Catherine of Sienna, Fabiola, Joan of Arc, Bernadette Soubirous, and Pierre Teilehard de Chardin. Not only in antiquity, but today as well, many are called to this path. However, it is difficult to recognize journeyers because many follow the inward journey in the midst of their normal life.

Spiritual journeying usually begins as the result of an awakening. In most instances the awakening involves a change based on input of new and conflicting information. Marilyn Ferguson (1980) suggests we change our minds through four possible routes. First, we can **change by exception**, which means our old belief system remains intact but allows for a handful of anomalies. Secondly, we can **change by increment**. We change bit by bit while not being aware we have changed. Then there is **pendulum change**, the abandonment of one closed and certain system for another. The fourth way of change is **paradigm change**, which involves transformation. It is this fourth dimension of change that allows information to come together in a new form or structure. It is within the process of the paradigm change that the spiritual journey occurs.

There are a number of additional factors that are relevant to the awakening of the state of consciousness that result in mind change. Some of these include societal or cultural conditioning, an independent natural predisposition to spiritual thinking, or an individual, transcendental experience through a connection a transformational group. Many cultural groups emphasize and encourage religious practice. However, for the most part it seems that individuals with a natural predisposition to spirituality or who have experienced paradigm-change thinking are the ones who hear, see, or feel something beyond the traditional religious rhetoric and move ahead to embark on their own personal spiritual journey.

Peace Pilgrim was a woman who in her midfifties disregarded her age, dropped her given name, and took on the name of her new profession, that which she professed to be, a Peace Pilgrim. From the first of January 1953 to her death in July 1981 she followed a vow: "I shall remain a wanderer until mankind has learned the ways of peace, walking until given shelter and fasting until given food" (Peace Pilgrim, 1983). She walked thousands of miles through the fifty states. She completed 25,000 miles in 1964 and at that point ceased counting. She looked like a silver-haired, suntanned, grandmother but had a radiant gaze and a joyful smile. She touched the lives of all whose path she crossed while sharing the message of peace wherever she trod.

Entry Point

The entry point of a spiritual journey may begin as a conscious, awakened decision. However, not all travelers begin the trip with lofty ideals and pure motives. There are many entry portals. People may begin the journey while in the midst of life's shadow. They are the ones who live in the "dark night of the soul," wrestling "the blue devil," or in their "cold winter's discontent." For these people the spiritual journey can begin at the bottom of the bottle, at the seeming end of the road, when they have no where else to go and no one left to whom they can turn.

Regardless of the portal of entry, all have the same opportunity. Each and every one of us has the capacity to undertake the journey requisite for healers, the journey of spiritual evolution. There are no necessary credentials, no prescribed paths, and no requirements. The only thing that is necessary is an open heart and mind and the willingness to risk and explore.

PURPOSE OF THE JOURNEY

The purpose of spiritual journeying is to foster and develop one's spiritual potential. Some may refer to this concept as developing or becoming conscious of your soul's purpose for this lifetime. During the journeying process maturation and individuation of the individual psyche should and usually do occur.

NATURE OF THE JOURNEY

Solitude

The nature of a spiritual journey requires that it be done in solitude. It is essentially a process of inner exploration, and the nature of inner work is that it be done alone. There are countless tales of those who withdrew from society to be alone on their spiritual quests. For example, Henry David Thoreau who spent a year at Walden Pond in Massachusetts, is remembered for writing a book and several treatises to describe his experiences. Initially he withdrew for external, political reasons, but his solitude awakened his inner spirit.

However, solitude does not necessarily require seclusion. Sometimes it is facilitated by involvement with others who are on a similar journey. Often participating in a group will awaken the participants or open their inner eyes by means of a heretofore unseen entry portal, made manifest by group synergy allowing the individual process to begin.

Regardless of the nature of the journey, it is important to take time to be still. Inspiration or insight does not usually strike a moving target: it only succeeds in striking another one where we might have been. It is the stillness that occurs in the solitude of deep self-reflection that allows us to hear our quiet, inner voice that best directs us on our journey.

Mode of Travel

The spiritual journey is an inward one and does not require physical travel. Some undertake this journey without ever leaving home. For the stay-at-home type or for those confined because of a physical limitation, the inner voice alone can clearly direct the journey. Stimulated solely by books, music, patio gardens, and/or an animal companion, some people may become advanced spiritual travelers. Theirs is an inner exploration within the confines of their own physical setting.

The outward spiritual traveler undertakes the same inward journey as the recluse but through the mode of physical space. Travel to unfamiliar places is a very effective means of stimulating our spiritual nature through the arousal of all the senses. In a new environment the sensory organs are bombarded with new sights, sounds, tastes, and aromas. These new external visions often induce the senses to accelerate the processing and translation of new information and experience into meaningful spiritual insights.

The mind is put to work analyzing and categorizing how things operate and how to function in a new setting. Likewise, the emotions are awakened in response to unfamiliar people, customs, culture, and language. With the physical, mental, and emotional domains awakened and alert, one's spiritual senses are also stimulated. Spiritual travelers are documented in Western literature in works such as Merton's *Seven Story Mountain*, Somerset Maugham's *The Razor's Edge*, Hilton's *Lost Horizon*, and the anonymous *Way of the Pilgrim*.

Time

If anything, the spiritual journey requires time. It is essential to create time for reflection and inner work and the solitude that they require. Consider the minimal twelve years that public law requires for basic, precollegiate, academic mental training. Or think about the Adepts of the Eastern traditions who invest large amounts of time in the seemingly simple act of meditation—a skill pursued to increase both inner and outer awareness. Consider athletes who train their bodies many hours every day in the pursuit of physical prowess. It follows that the spiritual journey undertaken to awaken and develop one's spiritual potential necessitates an investment of time.

A paradoxical aspect of time is that once spiritual journeying begins, it seldom concludes. One who enters this realm soon discovers that there are layers, on layers, on layers of new dimensions and new ways of perceiving. During the course of the inner work one discovers that each person is a manifestation of the pattern of consciousness of all that there is. Both the visible pattern of our bodies and the unseen pattern of our minds, feelings, and spirits are manifestations of a larger underlying pattern.

Being Open to the Flow of Spirit

To undertake a spiritual journey, one often leaves the familiar mental musings, including the physical surroundings as well, and paradoxically journeys both inward and outward. Journeys may be taken with specific goals in mind or with an open agenda and few expectations. The latter probably offers the opportunity for greater learning.

Although most people journey, it is through awakened consciousness or awareness and intent that the ordinary journey becomes a spiritual journey. For the traveler who has embarked on the spiritual journey with conscious intent and without delimiting expectations, the trip will inevitably be fruitful and much will be learned. From spiritual journeys one gains insight into the meaning and purpose of life and comes to better understand how the individual being is part of the whole process.

Retreat from the Distractions of the Temporal World

Sometimes life gets so complicated or busy that one needs to leave their everyday environment and go to setting befitting of fresh and new ideas. There are numerous retreat centers and guided retreat sessions that are available for the awakened participant. Once you are aware that these centers exist and particularly after participating in a retreat, awareness of additional opportunities increases. Often spiritual retreat centers are affiliated with churches or religious organizations. Within this structure guided retreats are held on a periodic basis ranging from half-day ventures to two-week or month-long intensive sessions. For those who are unfamiliar with this mode, a guided retreat is most valuable since the guide is knowledgeable in how to best lead the individual and/or group in the direction of the intended introspection.

Guided retreats are generally held in nature settings that are conducive to solitude and self-reflection. Many retreat centers are housed in wooded settings by a lake, river, or oceanside. In antiquity, water was believed to be a purifying vehicle, and most healing centers were located by bodies of water. Today, as in antiquity, an aesthetic setting is considered important during times of serious self-reflection or contemplation. The reason for this is twofold. First, if one is in transition, it is then important to be in a setting where your thoughts and sensibilities can be elevated and raised to visualize new possibilities. Secondly, centers of natural or artistic beauty stir the psyche toward affirmation and motivation to achieve the newly visualized possibilities. Thus you often emerge from guided retreats ignited with renewed zeal for new-found goals or directions.

In retreat settings you do not have to deal with temporal, worldly distractions that so often prevent us from quieting our minds and moving into deep relaxation. In addition, in retreat sites you are usually with others who are likewise on retreat for the purpose of self-reflection and personal growth. The energy generated by others in the same group joins with yours to create a heightened or intensified effect that may yield more powerful or significant insights.

Table 4-1
Tools to Promote Spiritual Growth

There are a variety of skills and techniques to help people on the journey. Some of these techniques are as follows:

- Self-reflection
- Meditation
- Prayer
- Dream journaling
- Individual and group retreats
- Psychological techniques
  Psychosynthesis
  Guided imagery
  Personal or group therapy sessions
- Travel
- Participating in transformational conferences and seminars

To illustrate with one example, during the reflective process one spends time contemplating personal questions such as the following:

- What is the meaning, purpose, and direction of my life?
- To what extent have I evolved on my life's journey?
- Am I achieving what I want to achieve in my life?
- What brings me pleasure, what causes me pain?
- Am I doing what brings me pleasure and satisfaction in life? If not, why not, and how can I change my situation?
- How are my values made operational in my day-to-day living?
- Can I become still enough to listen to the quiet inner voice that directs my being?
- How can I grow more fully?

It is through the consideration of such questions that one delves more deeply into the aspect of conscious living, and it is in living consciously that one engages in the spiritual journey.

END RESULT OF SPIRITUAL JOURNEYING

Regardless of what the nature of the spiritual journey has been, a weekend retreat, a trip around the world, or simply a period of reflective solitude, the end result is usually the same. One who makes a spiritual journey is never the same. Whether it is the result of active sensory bombardment or isolated inner work, you change. Both the senses and the mind are widened to new perceptions and possibilities. A whole new data bank of facts intertwine with spirit thus creating the ongoing evolution both for the individual and for our collective whole.

The end result of the journey is often reflected as action. An individual who has had a mind shift through the journeying process is the person who is inclined to assist others in their process by becoming a spiritual activist. Spiritually active people are both awakened and perceptive. Like the eagle they often soar silently until the optimal opportunity for prompt action is observed by their widely opened eyes. Then they act to assist others.

Many times a spiritually active person will guide or assist others through consistent, covert examples rather than more overtly obvious activism. Often people who are spiritually active lead lives of loving usefulness. You will not hear them protesting in crowds or asserting their beliefs from soapboxes. They are nevertheless spiritually active. They are the dedicated and loyal workers who honor and work hard for their employer, the volunteers who makes important things happen from behind the scenes, the parents who patiently nourish and raise children, the teachers who instill virtues and principles of honor in students, and the people who are there to lend a hand or offer support to their fellow brothers and sisters in times of need.

Spiritual activism is more than surface appearances such as religious persuasion and protestations of faith. It is the development of a sense of purpose and meaning in life that transcends the ordinary material world. It is coming to understand why we are here and what our mission is.

RELEVANCE TO HEALING

Healers must become aware of where they are on their own journeys to help others to begin or further facilitate their journeys. The healer guided by personal understandings can more easily facilitate the harmonious interconnectedness within and between persons, as well as with the interpersonal and physical environments and with the Ultimate Other or God as understood by the individual (Nagi-Jacobson and Burkhardt, 1989).

Accepting others as they are, where they are, without the traditional concern for defining, controlling, and changing, permits the spirit to expand and express itself. So many people have lived a life of control, definition, and judgment that the spirit has been driven far below the surface (Schunlior, 1989).

The healer is like a tuning fork through which the client or patient can begin to resonate with the consciousness of the universe. Entering a patient's room or walking through their front door, open and vulnerable, without definitions and judgements, is sometimes a charm sufficient to release the princess trapped within the fearful dragon (Rilke, 1962).

Once we journey, we recognize ourselves as part of the larger whole. As we integrate this awareness into our lives, our care becomes a noble service. We can rise to the occasion of living creatively, industriously, and wisely as we nurture the healing of others and serve as guides to those who are ready.

> **I slept and dreamt that life was joy,**
> **I woke and saw that life was service,**
> **I acted and behold, service was joy.**
>
> *Rabindranath Tagore*

Summary

Spiritual journeying involves a conscious decision to explore one's own inner self in relation to a larger cosmic consciousness. There is an awareness, gradual or abrupt, of the paradigm shift originating from sorting new and conflicting sets of information.

The sorting of the new information and experience affords the awakened individual the opportunity to enter through an entry portal to begin what can be a transformational process. The journeying process is done through inner work, often in solitude, with or without group support. Physical travel is often a part of the journey but not requisite to it. One who is engaged in spiritual journeying often emerges as a spiritual activist who covertly or overtly assists others in the healing process.

Healer Reflections

- Which changes have I experienced in my life that opened the possibility for my own spiritual journey?
- Am I aware of how the journey process relates to developing the inner light, a phenomenon common to many healers?
- Have I ever taken a symbolic spiritual journey?
- How would it feel to stay in a retreat center and focus on my spiritual life?

REFERENCES

Ferguson, M. *The aquarian conspiracy.* Los Angeles: J. P. Tarcher, 1980.

Nagai-Jacobson, M. G., & Burkhardt, M. A. Spirituality: Cornerstone of holistic nursing practice, *Holistic nursing practice,* 1989, *3*(3), 18–26.

Peace Pilgrim. Santa Fe: An Ocean Tree Book, 1983.

Rilke, R. M. *Letters to a young poet.* New York: Norton, 1962.

Schunlior, C. Nursing and the comic mask, *Holistic nursing practice.* 1989, *3*(3), 16.

Chapter 5

The Role of Intention

"For a person with a firm grasp of their intentions, neither the heated passions of their fellow-citizens ordaining something awful, nor the face of a tyrant before their very eyes, will shake their firm-based mind."

Horace (65–8 B.C.)

Empowering Yourself

Consider how it would feel to sincerely desire the best solution or outcome for the individual whose problems you will next attend.

Become aware of the danger of mistaking the use of your own psychological defense mechanisms for good intentions.

Schedule some time to practice focused intention on your own visions of health for yourself, a loved one, the community, and the planet.

Consider what the difference in your behavior would be if you believed that your intention alone without any other techniques or interventions made a difference in how someone felt.

DEVELOPING INTENTION

Most of us who chose the profession of nursing did so with intention. Not all of us had the intention to heal when we came to nursing, but certainly we all had some sense of calling. For most of us it was when we engaged in our practice that we began to understand the concept of intention.

Healing with Intention: Sandra's Story

Sandra was a nursing student. She was one of those who stayed at school during holidays to work extra to help pay for tuition. One hot night deep into the tiring summer, when the heat, the noise, and the inescapability of the city were overwhelming, she had a life crisis. Her insistent knocks woke her friend down the hall from a deep sleep. As she entered her friend's room, it was evident that she was in trouble. She had crude wrappings over her wrists. "It's just too terrible," she cried. "I just can't take it anymore, what am I going to do?" Her friend reacted immediately and responded to the emergency.

Ruth quickly dressed and told her what they were going to do together. Sandra allowed Ruth to take the lead as they walked across the street to the emergency room. Ruth spent the balance of the night with Sandra, first being present while her superficial wrist slashes were tended, and then during the long ordeal of getting her checked into the acute-care psychiatric division two blocks further down the street. It was a long, difficult night for them, yet Ruth knew with conviction and intention that she would see it through whatever it took. There was a specific reason to act and responsibility on her part to see it to conclusion.

Sandra ended up spending the better part of the following year in long-term rehabilitation. She rejoined the school the following year and eventually went on to become a nurse healer. She is an example of one who survived wounding and grew stronger as she learned from the experience. Ruth, who healed with intention at an early age, relished in her classmate's eventual accomplishments.

Observations

In this instance, and others like it, the healer knows when to act. Intention is strong and powerful and accomplishes known goals. There are times to act with intention and other times to be silent and allow the course of events to flow without interference.

TO HELP OR TO HEAL?—MISGUIDED INTENTIONS

There has been a growing tendency in recent years for many would-be healers, especially those schooled in the psychodynamic technique, to use the tactic of confrontation in their helping approach. It has become popular, for example, to talk in terms of addiction and codependency when considering almost any human problem, be it smoking, alcohol, caffeine consumption, eating, relationships, work, or personal motivation. On scrutiny, it appears the only area not addressed by this current addictive, codependency theory is breathing and elimination.

The following are some sample senarios from those "in recovery" who are attempting their own variety of helping intentions. John has been in therapy for six months working on his personal problems. He has been working on smoking cessation and has consequently also cut down on caffeine consumption. Sue's desk is next to John's at work and one day, unable to contain himself, he approaches her and with a confident smile says, "Hey Sue, that's your third cup of coffee today. Do you think you might have a caffeine addiction problem?" If you were Sue, how would you react?

In another example, it is Friday night, and Ted and Sue are out on a dancing date. They have been having a pleasant chat and Sue thinks maybe this relationship has possibilities. Ted, a member of Alcoholics Anonymous (AA) is drinking a coke. Sue has just finished a glass of white wine and answers affirmatively when the waitress asks if she would like another. Just then, Ted bends close, looks soberly at her, and declares, "Sue, I didn't know you had a drinking problem." How do you think Sue might react? How would you react?

There is an old saying that goes, "the road to hell is paved with good intentions," and although hell might not be the actual outcome, certainly healing is not either. It is the purity and clarity of the intention that we must scrutinize.

Because of the popularity of this theory, many people now believe they are either addicts, codependents, enablers, or some combination thereof. Once on the bandwagon of recovery, many become crusaders to have others join them. Thus, like John or Ted, they will confront almost anybody along their path. The projection of their particular, perceived diagnosis becomes like a banner. With some, the more people they confront, the more internally supported in their "recovery" process they become. It is as if the more people they can get to confess their problems of addictive or codependent patterns, the stronger the recovering addict feels inside. Confrontation of another's weakness actually does little for the other person and may in fact actually hurt the situation. The underlying subconscious motivation may more than likely be an attempt to stengthen the weak ego of the confronter.

It is important to remember that people are generally not ready to have your help unless they ask for it. When they ask for your advice or opinion, they indicate a readiness for help. Until that that time arrives, little can be accomplished by supposedly helpful confrontations.

Intentionality is subtle. Would-be healers must be careful about their intention to help others. What on the surface may feel like or seem to be good intention may in actuality be an internal issue being projected outward on another. Most of us use the psychological crutches of defense mechanisms at one time or another. Some use them frequently. They are used subconsciously to protect the ego when an individual does not have enough ego strength to accept the responsibility for their own thoughts or behavior. The most common defense mechanisms are rationalization (explaining something away), projection (projecting our own weaknesses, mistakes, or errors onto another), denial (refusal to accept our role in an event or problem), and repression (psychologically burying an issue that you are unable to deal with in the moment). These are common, albeit subconscious, techniques that most people use.

CULTIVATING AWARENESS OF OUR MOTIVATIONS

Growth is in an ever upward spiral. As we become increasingly conscious of our own behaviors, we are in a position to better understand ourselves. As we better understand ourselves, we can more clearly examine our real motivations in our intent to help others. It is with this incremental growth that we can begin to shed the defense mechanisms that served to protect us when we needed them and begin to move to a new level of maturity. It is with a strong ego that we are able to drop the defense mechanisms altogether and operate with pure, unclouded intention. When that occurs, one can begin to see without the haze of one's own problems obscuring the perceptions of the problems of another. Those endeavoring to help others must first help themselves. By becoming keenly aware of yourself, you work on and heal yourself as you endeavor to help others. It is through developing sensitivity that we learn about intentionality.

One who is serious about developing the attitudes and behaviors of a healer pays attention to the real motives behind the intention. A sensitive friend, caregiver, companion, or partner would, on most occasions, not be confrontive like John or Ted but would approach Sue in quite a different manner. Is it necessary for John or Ted to confront another in the first place? Is this truly helpful behavior, or is it in fact destructive behavior representing immaturity and misguided intentions. An important question one must ask before confronting others is, who am I really endeavoring to help—myself or another?

When I do workshops on developing awareness, one of my favorite photographic slides is a shell superimposed on a beautiful, empty beach at sunset. The caption says "Explore Inner Space." The next slide in the series depicts a single figure walking along the same beach at sunset. Its caption is simple and poignant; it says "Listen." I find these two pictures always capture the attention of the viewers. Something in the message is "right on." It is as if silence, solitude, reflection, and thought are the important elements required for the task of cultivating sensitivity. Once these initial working steps are taken, the real caring begins.

Once the reflective process is in progress, self-examination and introspection begin. This is the type of work that is done during the spiritual journey described in the last chapter. As the reflective process proceeds, ego strength is built. With a strong and secure ego one does not fall back on defense mechanisms that obscure the facts and block the pure intention requisite of healers.

THE HEALING POWER OF PRAYER

Prayer is perhaps one of the few forms of pure intention. When one engages in prayer, there are usually no ulterior motives and no need for defense mechanisms. One who prays usually communicates directly with God or a higher power so there is little need for self-deception since the request, thanks, or intent is moving away from the contracted, ego-shelled self into a greater dimension and greater purpose. The question I pose is, if prayer is an example of pure intention, does it work?

Researchers at Spindrift, an organization located in Oregon, used scientific methodology to study this very question (Owen, 1988). The way they answered the question was to conduct experiments. The one I found of particular interest was one done with sprouting seeds. In this experiment rye seeds were divided into two groups and planted in the same container with a string down the middle dividing the two groups into halves. Throughout the experiment the researchers watered and prayed for group A seeds and offered nothing but water to group B. The results were significant.

Consistently the group of seeds that were prayed for (group A) had a greater sprouting rate than did those not prayed for in group B. The Spindrift group went on to explore whether unhealthy seeds would still sprout with prayer. To answer this question they stressed the rye seeds by pouring salt water into the seed container, and then they prayed for them. This time the results were dramatic. The experimental group sprouts that were prayed for grew much better than before being stressed, indicating that prayer works better when the organism is unhealthy or under stress. This experiment is perhaps explained by the phenomenon of homeostasis: the greater the disharmony of an organism, the more quickly it will attempt to restructure to reestablish internal harmony. Both experiments affirm the healing power of pure intention as expressed through the mode of prayer.

THE PRAYER OF SAINT FRANCIS

This prayer is popular among nurse healers. It has even been put to music and sung at some healing conferences.

> Lord, make me an instrument
>   of your peace.
> Where there is hatred,
>   let me sow love.
> Where there is injury, pardon.
> Where there is doubt, faith.
> Where there is despair, hope.
> Where there is darkness, light,
>   and where there is
>   sadness, joy.
> O Divine Master, grant that
>   I may not so much seek
>   to be consoled, as to console;
> To be understood,
>   as to understand;
> To be loved, as to love;
> For it is in giving that we
>   receive—
> It is in pardoning that we are
>   pardoned;
> And it is in dying that we are
>   born to eternal life.

THE DIFFERENCE BETWEEN HOPE AND INTENTION

Is there a difference between hope and intention, and does it matter which term we use? In many instances people will say such things as, "I sure hope I can do this," or "I hope I succeed," or "I hope he gets home all right." Generally the word hope is a loosely defined, vague term that is generally immeasurable and as such is usually likewise unachievable. Intent, on the other hand, is capable of being clearly defined, visualized, and therefore actualized. When one says, "I intend to accomplish such and such," there is often an accompanying mental picture of just what steps will be involved to actually achieve the result. With intention one takes the stance of responsibility and formulates action steps to achieve the desired intention. Intention, a word of power and action, is essential of all who would be healers.

Healer Reflections

- Am I aware of my defense mechanisms that may be blocking the opening of my pure intention for healing?
- Are there times in my life when I have pure intention to help another?
- Do I understand how healing can flow through me based solely on my pure intentions when I act as a clear channel without subconscious blocks and interferences?

REFERENCE

Owen, R. *Qualitative research: The early years* Salem, Oreg.: Greyhaven Books, 1988.

Chapter 6

Recovery From Wounding

"Wash what is dirty, water what is dry, heal what is wounded. Bend what is stiff, warm what is cold, guide what goes off the road."

Archbishop Stephen Langton

Empowering Yourself

Note how healers have both strengths and weaknesses.

Consider that during the journey of each healer, at least once, and often many times, the shadow must be faced. It is in facing one's own personal shadow, going into the fire, that new strength is born.

Understand the significance of woundedness.

Learn methods to heal your wounds.

WOUNDING

Wounding takes many forms and has many faces. Physical wounding may be as mundane as a bout of the common cold or as traumatic as a spinal cord injury. Mental wounding could be a setback from a failed college examination or as profound as mental retardation. Spiritual wounding, as other types of wounding, can range the gamet from simple to complex. A wounding must be recognized for healing to begin.

Jimmy—A Contemporary Healer

Jimmy was a urology patient on the surgical ward where he was admitted for obstruction of his one remaining kidney. He was 44 years old now, but at the age of 19 he dived into a shallow pool and sustained a neck injury that rendered him quadriplegic. He had some limited use of his hands but was otherwise unable to do anything for himself. He had to be turned, dressed, fed, toileted, and bathed by others. He had been incapacitated in this condition for 25 years.

The thing about Jimmy that was heroic was his attitude.One day when I arrived to dress his open, decubitus ulcers and clean his catheter drain, I was visibly upset about another matter, something that had nothing to do with Jimmy. I was rushing around and obviously preoccupied with a previous problem. When I glanced at him, I noticed his concerned expression. As I began my work, I apologized about my previous preoccupation and he replied, "I know you are so busy. The work you do is difficult. Do you know that I pray for you? I hope things will be easier for you soon." Immediately I realized that Jimmy was attempting to help me. Sure, I was doing the dressing change, but it was his reaching out to me that began the dialogue between us. As we talked, the atmosphere noticeably softened, and the charged state of activity I was in when I entered changed to reflect his peaceful mood.

Jimmy's family had cared for him for 25 years. They had learned the give and take of the reciprocal relationship. They tended his wounds, and he returned all he could with his attitude of gratitude and love. He had worked long and hard on developing forgiveness of himself, for his recklessness, and the world for allowing it to happen. He had come to peace with himself and gave on any occasion whatever he could, and what he gave was the peace of himself and encouragement to those who came to him within the confines of his physical environment.

I did not see Jimmy after our last dressing change. He was scheduled for surgery the following morning. Apparently there was difficulty with the procedure, and he died on the operating-room table.

Observations

Healers are not always who we initially think they are. Sometimes the healer is the nurse, and sometimes it is the practicing nurse's client or nurse educator's student. The joy, however, is that all of us have the qualities it takes to become healers. Sometimes it is just necessary to recognize these qualities within ourselves and then to mold and shape or heal them for us to become the finest kind of person—a nurse healer.

SIGNIFICANCE OF WOUNDEDNESS

At one time or another, in one way or another, each of us has been wounded. For some, such as Jimmy above, it may have been a physical wound; for others it may have been through another mode such as child abuse, illness, or abandonment. Woundedness is not always overtly apparent. I have known healers who have been painfully wounded yet, because they still lack the strength to see it, fail to perceive it. Then there are others who during their life processes transcended their woundedness without ever consciously addressing it. Even though they may not have consciously faced their woundedness, it is there. Those healers who have not recognized their woundedness and became excellent healers anyway probably did so because, at least to some extent, they still use the open wounds to activate and utilize the healing channel.

Other healers, however, who do not recognize their woundedness or refuse to investigate its possibility, may in fact hide from the truth. One of the many remarkable things about our bodies is the capacity they have to harbor, carry, and hide wounds within them. The difficulty is that, paradoxically, we really have nowhere to hide them. We are such complex, biopsychosocial creatures that in one way or another, in one place or another, our unhealed woundedness will surface. In one person past hurts may be masked in psychological or emotional difficulties, while in another the wound may mainifest in physical symptoms or disease, and in still another there may be repeated problems with relationships.

Most people do recognize their hurts. They may be repressed or suppressed for some time, but when an opportunity comes for unearthing and processing woundedness, the memories usually rush to the surface, begging to be attended. No one likes to bear the weight of carrying the burden of unhealed wounds, but unfortunately many do.

Social Support

Some of our hurts seem so severe that we think we cannot share them with anyone else. We think no one could understand the brokenness of our body, mind, and spirit. Yet as we listen to hundreds of stories of woundedness of contemporary healers, we come to understand that each story, although poignant and unique in itself, fits into the collective of archetypical woundedness.

RECOVERY FROM WOUNDEDNESS

The experience of being in the figurative wilderness is a state from which we seek relief. When we have suffered long enough, we want out. It is at this time that many begin to strive for maturity and wisdom. Through the course of the healing journey each of us has the capacity to emerge as a hero or heroine by becoming more fully human and simultaneously more godlike or goddesslike.

The Light and the Shadow

Human life contains polarity, and polarity implies opposition. For example, polarities include such concepts as light/dark, masculine/feminine, hot/cold, and right/wrong. In polarity there is the light (white), the shadow (black), and all the shades of grey between most issues. The majority of issues and their resolution are seldom black or white but instead are usually found within the grey area. Love, service, and empowerment lie within the area of light, while tragedy, pain, and wounds reside within the shadow. The earth has opposing poles, as do certain mechanical devices such as the magnet. Just as a magnet cannot be a magnet without an opposite to attract it, so too do humans require polarities. Without the light we have no concept of the shadow, and without the shadow we cannot appreciate the light. The contrast is essential (Dossey, 1988).

Facing the Shadow

One way to conceive of health is to know suffering. A primary way we can really develop and emerge as healers is to have first-hand experience in healing our own pain. The shadow may be physical illness or emotional pain; it may be broken relationships or spiritual ennui. Whatever it is, it must be faced before we become healers. We cannot become whole unless and until we face the whole. Too often people skim across the surface, going from peak to peak, person to person, without taking the act of courage it demands to step back and begin an indepth exploration of the dark side of one's own shadow. Moving from one relationship to another is one example of how individuals shield themselves from looking inward. It is easier to blame the problem on someone else than to walk into your own shadow and look for solutions there. Yet, that is where most real solutions lie.

Whatever the problem, the pattern of it will recur again and again, in different forms, until it is squarely faced and finally dealt with. It is when we deny a problem and repress it subconsciously that it has the potential to cause psychological, physical, or relationship problems. When a major, stress-causing event occurs, the easiest thing to do is to repress the meaning of the darkness. Yet, over time the consequences of the failure to understand this meaning will surface again. At some point we must address the shadow and examine our wounds. We must identify our weaknesses, as well as recognize and develop our strengths. It is only when we face and heal the shadow that we allow a powerful healing dimension of our personality to be born. Without healing, or channeling our wounds into healing conduits, there is little chance of emerging with the strength to heal others.

When going into their own shadow some people have episodes similar to the near death experience (NDE). In the NDE people who have had clinical deaths and recover give reports of traversing forward through a tunnel of brilliant white light. They feel a previously unexperienced joy of connection with a higher consciousness and a greater purpose in living following recovery. When facing their psychological shadow some individuals report a parallel experience, but this time the tunnel is dimly lit and covered with thorns. However, when traveling into it far enough they can see answers and solutions at the other end. Sometimes this image comes in dreams, sometimes during the depths of despair, but this is the image some report.

THE WOUNDED HEALER

Some of the current problems our society faces are probably the result of not facing the shadow of our individual and collective woundedness. Many nurses entered the profession because of conscious or unconscious recognition of their own woundedness. Unfortunately, most are probably unconscious of their maladies, but in seeking to help others they are unconsiously looking for ways to help themselves. The psychological defense mechanism of projection allows caregivers to see in another what is actually inside themselves. Nurses working through this defense mechanism are actually trying to help themselves as they project healing energies onto others.

Also noteworthy is the fact that the thrust of most academic nursing programs involves an outwardly directed approach. The emphasis is on learning facts and techniques and on applying these skills outward to clients. Little, if any, attention is given during the formative professional years to being inward bound. However, it is this inward, personal exploration that results in significant, if not essential, understanding of who we really are. Before we embark on the journey of healing, we must first heal our own wounds and garner our own resources to learn how to heal ourselves. Without facing our own individual and collective wounds we will only misguidely project our hurts onto others.

Of course, self-healing is a lifelong process. Just because we emerged healed from one crisis does not mean we will have completed the recovery work. As long as we live, we will continue to have unexpected challenges. They are probably given to us as continuing opportunities to build our character and develop wisdom.

Empowerment Through Recovery

Healing is a mysterious event that occurs from a source or in a way that our minds cannot yet comprehend. It is related to inspiration, a taking in of the spirit. True we have technological marvels, pharmaceutical aids, and surgical measures that cure pathophysiological, cellular-based, physical illness, but is this healing or curing? There are thousands of documented cases of miraculous healings that occur frequently in shrines, temples, and churches throughout the world. There are spontaneous reversals of terminal cancers, unsighted people with unexplained restored vision, cripples who walk again, and those who come to peace with themselves and others before the transition of the physical body into the realm of death. What causes these occurrences? Is it because of interventions of the actions of a person known as healer, or is it the connection with a greater phenomenon from within or without stimulated by faith or some other reality?

Let us examine the process. It is the openness of an individual that makes for vulnerability, and it is through vulnerability that we can become wounded. When wounded in any fashion we have the potential for closing, becoming embittered and hardened, or the potential for opening the psyche. It is through the open psyche that healing energy has the capacity to flow. Pain, if consciously channeled, can serve to help an individual get in touch with powers greater than their ego and to become aware of the conduit through which the mysterious healing energy flows. It is by healing ourselves and transcending our wounds that we have the potential to become healers. It is when we offer our suffering up to a higher source that we enter the coredemptive process. In this process the consciousness of our suffering may be pooled into the collective unconscious, serving to offset and temper other events within the context of the whole of the human condition. Through a conscious awareness of personal suffering, there is the opportunity to learn compassion, forgiveness, and love, the attributes of a true nurse healer.

Is there a correlation between the relationship of one who suffers and the healer? More than likely there is a correlation between wounding, healers, and the occurrence of healing. Those who consciously serve as healers have opened a channel within themselves through which healing energy can flow. The healing does not come from them but rather through them as through a conduit. The relationship between wounding and the flow of this phenomenon has to do with the openness of the healer. To most healers it does not matter whether they are healed but whether they emerge from the wounding process as healers of others. In some instances it may be that the openness of their unhealed wound is what allows the conduit to remain open.

HEALING THE WOUNDS

Without complete recovery by channeling of the wound into healing or other forms of creativity, problems develop. Those who do not use their pain to create a conduit healing channel or to sublimate the energies into creative pathways stand the risk of developing bitterness, disillusionment, or hostility. This neither aids the wounded one nor facilitates the journey along the path to becoming a healer of others. Table 6-1 outlines steps to heal recognized wounds.

Table 6-1
Healing the Wounds

Open awareness to the fact that wounding has occurred.

Make a mental commitment to address the problem.

Set aside time to explore the issue(s).

Take definitive steps to heal the wound.
   Journaling
   Therapy/counseling
   Dream work
   Other steps

We all know of those who have been wounded with some unfortunate result: the abused daughter who cannot forgive her father, the divorcee who hates all men, or the alcoholic turned mean. When working with ourselves or with others who have handled their wounding in this way, there are steps that can be taken to remedy the situation. First, there must be an awareness of the fact that wounding has occurred. This in itself is not always readily apparent or necessarily easy to discover. However, when this awareness surfaces, there must be some sort of commitment made on the part of the individual for introspection, a time set aside to mentally return to the time of wounding, and definitive steps taken to heal the wound.

Psychosynthesis, psychotherapy, dream work, journaling, and involvement with a religious group and/or support groups are some ways that old wounds can be healed within an established supportive environment. Each of these modalities is in itself a developed form of healing therapy, and each requires a knowledgeable professional guide. When wounds are treated in this fashion, the pain of the event is recalled, yet the environment has changed, and new support networks have been established. This allows the wound to be examined and healed in a supportive atmosphere that was probably absent when the wounding initially occurred.

It is never too late to heal an old trauma. For example, it is often in middle age that adults discover dynamic techniques that help heal the wounded inner child. Trauma that occurred during the first 10 years of life can be, and has been for many, recalled and healed during the adult experience. People who have undergone this therapy report a tremendous sense of release of burdens, which they were not even aware they had been carrying, and a renewal in their zest for living.

Personal and collective empowerment comes from healing wounds and developing strengths. Individually we are increasingly balanced and more effective. Collectively, as more of us reflect stability and joy, our society can become increasingly secure and more energies can be placed in areas of growth and evolution instead of in continual crisis intervention.

DEVELOPING SKILLS
FOR SELF-HEALING

There are a variety of skills and actions one can utilize to hasten the healing process.

Time

We must not discount time's importance, for even the most painful wounds heal through the mode of time.

Verbal Expression

Healing comes from active communication of the pain. Expressing the hurt somehow always softens it. In the sharing process of speaking with a trusted friend, therapist, or special support group of others we can usually dissipate the trapped energy of emotional pain. Someone else can help diffuse the acuity of our suffering by listening, mirroring, and/or offering supportive feedback.

Written Expression

Written expression through the modes of journaling, dream analysis, or various forms of art can be very valuable. In this mode the content does not need to be shared with another. The simple reflecting by the writer usually aids in understanding the crisis event.

Physical Exertion

Physical exercise is another form of acting out and lessening pent up feelings. Many people find regular physical exercise as beneficial as psychotherapy and certainly much less expensive.

Service

Another effective and valuable way to heal ourselves is by turning our focus outward. There are times when we have done all we can possibly do and still there is no way to reverse the situation or stop the pain. We all know of parents whose children have died, spouses lost through death or divorce, or countless other tragic episodes. At times like these there is little benefit from looking inward. There is not much that can be yielded from within when there is so much emptiness. Therefore, at times like this, there may be more benefit in moving the focus away from one's self to another.

Barbara Bush, First Lady and wife of former United States President George Bush, tells a story of returning from two years in China and suffering a serious depression. When discovering that inward work yielded nothing other than more depression, she tried another approach and launched full steam into volunteer work. It was her work with charity that was her saving grace and turned her life around. Later when her three-year-old child died, it was again her nonstop volunteer work caring for the hospitalized that kept her going and brought her through another potentially serious depression.

When we become aware that there are always those who are worse off than we, this idea alone can often get us through even the hardest of times and help us recover from the most difficult wounding. There are times in most people's lives when the most effective cure may be caring for those who are less fortunate than they are.

Reclaiming Our Power

Another strategy is the notion of reclaiming our own personal power for full recovery. During times of emotional wounding what often happens is that we have given our power to another. We must become stronger by learning to reclaim our own dissipated personal power. The greatest source of strength is within and from attunement with the channel of power available to us from higher guidance. When we reconnect with these powers, we are then on the path of healing.

Health and healing can be conceived of as an ever upward spiral. It does not end when we have healed one wound, for another surely awaits us. Patterns will be repeated until we learn the meaning of the messages they attempt to give us.

THE FOUR PHASES OF HEALING

Healing from any type of wounding involves four distinct phases. The first is the **reaction** to the situation that occurred. In a physical wound there will be inflammation around the wound site and fever to fight infection. In emotional wounding there may be arguments and tears. Similar to physical wounding, there is an initial shock and intense pain that claims one's attention and totally shatters one's equilibrium. There is a flood of emotion, which may be thought of as psychologically analogous to physical bleeding.

The second component of healing is **regeneration**. On the physical plane, cells and tissues begin the remarkable reconstruction process. Eventually scabs form and scar tissue fills in the wound site. On an emotional level grieving occurs. Gradually the hurt is diminished, and the pain recedes into the recesses of subconsciousness.

The third phase of healing is **adaptation**. Physically one may learn to walk with a limp, "see" through the fingers with braille, or eliminate through a colostomy bag. Adaptation occurs when one can return to the routine of daily life without the pain of constant distraction. Both physical and emotional wounds may ache on occasion for years to come but not to the point of the initial disequilibrium.

Real recovery comes in the fourth phase of **empowerment**. Through the work done in the recovery process one may actually become stronger and wiser. Most individuals who have made great contributions to our world have evolved from the fighting back and recovery of the tragedy of their own personal wounding.

One who would become a healer must first understand the mysterious connection between illness and health. Healing power not only flows through those who know wellness but more importantly through those who have been ill or known the darkness of the shadow and have been healed. For the most part, people in whom the healing power moves will be those who have come in contact with their own wounds and have lived through the process of healing.

Healer Reflections

Am I aware of my strengths and weaknesses? Name them.

Have I faced my shadow? Do I understand the importance of doing so? Do I take the necessary time and do I have some form of support to help me tend my wounds?

What phase am I in in my own personal healing process?

What am I doing to heal my wounds?

REFERENCES

Dossey, B. Nurse as healer. In Dossey, B., Keegan, L., Guzzetta, C. & Kolkmeier, L. (aus.) *Holistic nursing: A handbook for practice.* Gaithersburg, MD: Aspen Publishing, 1988.

Peck, S. M. *The road less traveled.* New York: Simon and Schuster, 1978.

Snow, C. & Willard, D. *I'm dying to take care of you.* Redmond, Wash.: Professional Counselor Books, 1989.

Weil, A. *Health and healing.* Boston: Houghton Mifflin Company, 1983.

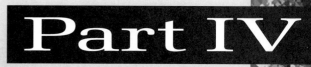

Part IV

Embracing Healing Attitudes

ATTITUDE

The longer I live, the more I realize the impact of attitude on life. Attitude, to me, is more important than facts. It is more important than the past, than education, than money, than circumstances, than failures, than successes, than what other people think or say or do. It is more important than appearance, giftedness, or skill. It can make or break a hospital, a nursing unit, or a home. The remarkable thing is that we have a choice every day regarding the attitude we will embrace for that day. We cannot change the past . . . we cannot change the fact that people will act in a certain way. We cannot change the inevitable. The only thing we can do is play on the one given we have, and that is our attitude. . . . I am convinced that life is 10% what happens to you and 90% how you react to it. And so it is with all of us. . . . we have a choice about our attitude.

by Charles Swindoll
(modified by Lynn Keegan)

Chapter

7

Attunement With the Natural World

"We are made one with Nature; there is heard His voice in all her music, from the moan of thunder, to the song of night's sweet bird.

Shelley (1792–1822)

Empowering Yourself

Consider how contact with nature relates to the ability to heal.

Think of some special place that you can go to strengthen your connection with the natural world.

Know that by attuning to the natural world we can learn to transform burdensome problems into passing nuisances on the path of life.

Learn the relationship of dreaming to healing.

THE FAST-PACED TECHNOLOGICAL WORLD

At least once, and usually two or three times each year, I journey to an environment where I can cloister away from the modern, fast-paced world and return to a simple way of living for a week or so. For me, like most people, it is not easy to accomplish this feat of getting away. The questions one might pose are how can we, why should we, and why would we want to abdicate our worldly roles and responsibilities to retreat and live in an ascetic manner? What does attunement with the natural world have to do with becoming a healer?

Almost everyone who is born today, at least in America, arrives into a fast-paced, technological society. Sophisticated, automated processes regulate even the miracle of birth. Most people, for most of their lives, spend their time engaged within a mechanized culture. It seems the more immersed we are individually and collectively, the more regulated, clock-oriented, and analytical we become. Conversely, much of the healing process is natural and mysterious and related to a connection with divinity. This connection can be quickened by attunement with the natural world. When one lives in the midst of nature, alignment with the basic process of an inborn, spiritual order begins within the human psyche.

In one of his most popular sonnets, William Wordsworth lamented that

> The world is too much with us; late and soon
> Getting and spending, we lay waste our powers:
> Little we see in Nature that is ours . . .

Henry David Thoreau, a mid–nineteenth century philosopher, addressed the problem of too much crowding and noise over 100 years ago by building a cabin by a quiet pond in Massachusetts. He lived in it for two years in relative solitude, studying nature, thinking, writing, and examining his thoughts. During this period he kept a journal that grew into the book *Walden,* a classic of American literature. The essence of his philosophy is that all of us need reflective time.

It does not matter which natural environment the contemporary nurse chooses. The seashore, the desert, the high plains, the deep forest, the pristine polar arctic, the jungle, or just an old-fashioned family farm will suffice. An environment ruled by natural rhythms, one without electricity, highways, and most conveniences to which we have grown so accustomed, is very helpful in awakening and restoring the sensitivities so necessary to becoming a healer. When one consciously lives within an environment of natural rhythms, there is an opportunity to resonate with the mysterious spiritual powers of healing. When you become part of the process of the ebb and flow of nature, it is easier to understand the ebb and flow of illness and healing. You develop heightened sensitivities and respect for the process simply by observing and coparticipating with the flora and fauna, the insects and spiders, the elements of weather in the wild, the beginning and end of natural days, and the dark mystery of the mechanically unaided night. When you become immersed in these natural rhythms, subtle sensitivities develop. The development and awareness of your relationship to the natural world is one aspect of your evolution as a healer.

CREATING THE SPACE/TIME FOR ATTUNEMENT

How can you, in the midst of life's busyness, find these opportunities for excursions into the natural world? There are actually numerous unrecognized opportunities for this experience. One reason we do not identify many chances is because often our immersion in the technological milieu dulls our sensitivities to the possible. External noise and busyness lessen our chance of hearing the inner voice of guidance. Because of this we narrow our perception of the possibility of a wider range of experience. There is, however, easy access to the natural world. Often it is as close as our own backyard. Table 7-1 lists ways anyone can enhance their connection with mother Earth.

Table 7-1
Ways to Increase Your Connection with the Natural World

Cultivate a vegetable or flower garden.
Begin a compost pile.
Plant trees and watch them grow.
Visit parks or natural areas at least once a month.
Take a job as a summer-camp nurse.
Go on early morning walks as the sun rises.
Take late night walks under starry, summer skies.
Keep a potted, growing plant in your work area.
Make ongoing, daily mental notes about the colors, characteristics, and feelings of whatever season you are currently experiencing.

Lie in an open meadow and listen to the wind.
Open your windows and fill your work and living space with
natural light and fresh air.

Once separated from the rush and busyness of the modern technological world, removed from television, radios, newspapers, automobiles,
and other worldly distractions, what happens, and why is it important
to becoming a nurse healer? When one retreats and refreshes their
being, there is a concomitant increase in sensitivity. Sensitivity is part
of the individuation process. It is this process that enables us to further understand and express the process of healing.

Remember Wordsworth's phrase, "The world is too much with us." It is
possible to overwork or overuse a particular part of the mind in just the
same way that we wear out a pair of shoes. The difference, however,
between the living cells of our being and inanimate articles is that we
cannot mend the holes in the soles of our shoes by putting them aside,
but the tired parts of our body-mind-spirit can be rested and restored.

There are many ways to overcome the worry and mental strain that
accompanies the life of a nurse healer. One of these ways is through a
change of environment and a change of pace. When we use this
method of healing, we must be aware that even though we change our
place we still have constant mind chatter. Consequently, when you
select a pastoral change, remember to refocus mental thinking. In the
beginning try to direct thinking to a task related to the natural environment. Some suggestions are as follows:

- Plan, prepare for, and go camping in a national park.
- Put up a tent and go for a family outing in your own backyard.
- Collect stones and build an outdoor cookout pit.
- Look for objects from nature and arrange an indoor centerpiece
  for a table.
- Build your own or join with your extended family or neighbors to
  build a week-end or summer retreat.

The idea is to create a mental focus to exercise other areas of your
mind. When doing this, the mental areas that have been overworked
can rest as mental activity is redirected into new receptors.

When we master the art of quieting the mind and attuning to the natural world, we are able to release or transform burdensome cares and
concerns allowing them to become but transitory nuisances on the
path of life.

In natural settings we experience the fact that we are not separate beings, but all inexorably interrelated. We are able to live, to unfold, and to "become" because the environment sustains us. Living close to the earth humbles and fills you with gratitude for all the universal elements that support life. In the wild you come to appreciate the delicate balance of life and learn that we need all the creatures. We become increasingly grateful for all the animals and insects, flora and fauna, the stars and the stones, for all beings and their works. In nature one learns that there is no randomness but rather that all is interrelated. Thus by becoming attuned to the natural world we develop the important and necessary attitudinal sensitivities of becoming effective healers. It is when we give thanks for these fresh insights that we acknowledge our place in the universe and become open to dimensions beyond the personal.

DREAMING AND HEALING

A few thoughts here on dreaming seem appropriate. Often when we attune to a natural environment, we have the capacity to awaken or expand our dreaming. It is perhaps not so necessary to dwell on the interpretation of your dreams as it is to precondition them. It is possible to condition dreams in such a way that they bring healing. Dreams may actually be a portal to alternate spaces. If this is the case, it is likewise important to realize that not all of these spaces are beneficial to the healing process. One must attempt to tune the dreaming faculties of the subconscious into the very highest forms of existence. To become a healer it is necessary to align our conscious and subconscious thoughts with peace, harmony, and tranquility. Dreaming then becomes critical to the centering process. Going into the dreaming process is akin to going into a maze with all sorts of alternate pathways that lead to dead ends and possible horrific endings. One is better equipped by first studying the map of the maze and programming the subconscious mind into the paths of life, light, peace, harmony, tranquility, and love. One does this by having positive, loving thoughts, following the prayer process, listening to gentle music, or going through progressive relaxation before sleeping (all of these techniques are discussed in Section VI of this book). The thought process must be centered and focused, not diffused and troubled.

The following exercise described in Table 7-2 has worked for many. Practice it and see how it works for you.

Table 7-2
Twelve Step Self-Programming Exercise for Cultivation of Healing Dreams

1. Turn off the television, radio, or other mechanical devices at least a half hour before bedtime.

2. If possible attune your consciousness to the sounds and sensations of nature during the evening.
   - Note the birds bedding chorus
   - Listen to the insects on warm summer evenings
   - Become aware of how the breeze decreases at sunset

3. Spend a few minutes journaling your day's activities and impressions.

4. Mentally review your accomplishments of the day and consider how you might have altered outcomes.

5. Dwell for a moment on loving kindness and forgiveness of yourself and others with whom you interacted today.

6. Decide to put aside differences with others and to gently come to closure on this day.

7. Open your awareness to the immensity of the cosmos. Mentally feel your own protected place in the universe.

8. Feel a sense of connection with all brethren life-forms.

9. Begin to allow one issue of present concern to surface to your conscious mind.

10. Begin to place this issue within the framework of universal consciousness.

11. Ask for answers or solutions as you sleep and dream.

12. On awakening remember your previous night's request and allow the answers to your petition to surface.

Bedtime Ritual

In the days before television and technology, parents use to rock and sing their children to sleep. The rocking stimulated the neurolinguistic feeling process. The voice, melody, and rhythm all led to a tranquil, serene, and secure dream process that facilitated the body, mind, and spiritual development of the child. This was a significant part of the nurturing and healing process for the child.

As an adult if you want to heal yourself, then consider this old, time-tested ritual of music, rhythm, and relaxation before sleeping. All who would become healers should profit from creative dreaming. Try to establish a relaxing bedtime ritual to allow your dreams and nighttime, subconscious, problem-solving processes the opportunity to open and actuate.

When one is in the process of becoming a healer, it is done from multiple planes of reality. Popular spiritual and transformational authors Castanedas, Andrews, and MacLaine all described the process of "becoming" in terms of storytelling. The staging ground from which they operate is from a different level of reality. Some call it magic, but these authors describe it as getting in touch with the higher and/or deeper aspects of yourself by entering into another plane of existence. The portals described in their popular books included ritual ceremonies, isolation, and expectation. All occurred in areas of seclusion from the technological world.

An attitude of respect and appreciation for the natural world is one of the characteristics of healers. As you reflect on this chapter, consider ways you can strengthen your appreciation for and attunement with nature's bounty.

Healer Reflections

When was my last immersion into the natural world?

Do I believe it is important to strengthen my ties with nature?

What does being in the natural world mean to or do for me?

Do I use dreaming in a self-healing manner?

Chapter

Joy and Empowerment Through Service

"I don't know what your destiny will be, but one thing I know; the only ones among you who will be truly happy are those who will have sought and found how to serve."

Albert Schweitzer

Empowering Yourself

Identify with the nurse in the first story and try to understand how she can become empowered, as well as empower others, through her service.

Acknowledge the value of a joyful disposition when dealing with others.

Observe how a joyful disposition serves to enable another to garner their own healing resources during times of crisis.

JOY AND EMPOWERMENT

When we consider the topic of joy and empowerment through service, the questions that come to mind are, whose joy and whose empowerment? The answer gratifyingly is that both the server and the served are empowered. Anytime service is performed from an awakened, conscious sense, there is an opportunity for positive attitudes and behaviors to ensue. Although we still do not have scientific instrumentation to measure it, there are probably positive electrons or energies generated from positive thoughts and actions. Hence when we function with joy we are a conduit for forces of empowerment.

Miranda's Story

Miranda was excited but apprehensive; this was her first evening on pediatrics. As she made her way down the hall for report she witnessed a loud, combative four-year-old boy with multiple facial deformities being restrained by an irritated man, probably the boy's father. The child threw his monstrous head back and forth as drool and incoherent speech flowed from his gaping mouth. His wide set, puffy eyes met hers and his face moved into a grimacelike grin. "Please God, not me," Miranda voiced to herself. "Please don't let this child be assigned to me. There are plenty of children here tonight. I'll gladly take care of anyone else, just not this one. Please, God." She entered the nurses' station and looked at her assignment, "Oh, no." Her plea had not been heard; he was hers for the next eight hours. A flair of annoyance rushed her, how could the charge nurse do this? Why me, she continued to reflect, and how can I get through this shift?

During report Miranda heard more. Not only did Jerome have multiple facial anomalies, but he was also retarded, on seizure precautions, had to be spoon-fed, and needed a specimen for urine culture and sensitivity.

Another nurse smiled across the report table and said, "Welcome to pediatrics. We take turns with Jerome, if you need help just holler—we all know him."

"Thanks," Miranda replied while gritting her teeth, wondering if she would survive the evening.

Her first job was to meet the child and introduce herself to the dad. Then she had to take Jerome's vital signs and give his medications.

She took a deep breath and headed into his room. "Hello, Mr. M. I'm Jerome's nurse."

"Hey girl, I'm glad to see you," Dad responded. "Okay, I'm outta here. Here buddy." With that he thrust the writhing child into her arms and took off.

Color mounted in Miranda's face as her arms supported the wiggling boy while his drool flowed down the bodice of her new uniform. Tears welled in her eyes as Jerome's arms flailed aimlessly against unseen adversaries. "Why me, God, why me?" Miranda voiced in her mind.

The evening hours advanced as Miranda did one task at a time. Slowly and methodically she cleaned him, fed him, medicated him, and obtained a urine specimen. At bedtime she even attempted to rock him but to no avail. He only threw his head back and forth, arched his crooked back, and screeched incoherently. Finally, while he lay prone in his crib, the bedtime chloral hydrate took effect and his agitation melted into sleep. Silently, Miranda lifted her hand from his back, adjusted his covers, and gratefully exited Jerome's room.

At 9 P.M. she crumpled into a chair at the desk and began to chart. "Hey, Miranda, you've got the makings of a good pediatric nurse. Five straight hours of Jerome and you didn't ask for help once. Way to go," said the nurse she had met in report.

"Tell me, Samantha, is it always this hard?"

Suddenly the ward clerk turned toward the nurses, "Who is Jerome's primary nurse?"

"I am," Miranda meekly replied.

"It's his Dad, he wants to talk to his nurse," the clerk said.

"Miranda took the call as she thought to herself, "What now?"

"Hi nurse, how's the kid?" a coarse voice boomed from the receiver.

"Jerome is sleeping now. He had his dinner, a bath, and plenty of activity."

"Thanks nurse. I'll be back tomorrow after work. See ya then."

Observations

Through this story we see how Miranda serves first because of duty or obligation. However, it is through this service that she begins to realize the empowerment she has even on her very first shift of work. If she learns to recognize this ability and becomes increasingly conscious of the concept, she is then on her way to becoming a nurse healer.

Jane and Sam

Jane smartly slapped the syringe, pushing the plunger in an exacting fashion to flip out the single, remaining air bubble as she held the small, calibrated tube high between her eyes and the ceiling light. She softly whistled a simple tune as she did this procedure so automatic to her now. She swiftly turned toward Sam and said, "pull your britches down now and roll over, this will just take a moment. Great, now take a deep breath. This will feel like a bee sting." With a quick, decisive movement she thrust the syringe deep into the gluteal muscle and with firm thumb-pressure plunged the liquid medication into his body. The needle was out and discarded in the Sharps container before Sam could say ouch. He turned toward her and she was mock dancing with empty, upturned hands waving in the air and her whistle replaced by a jazzy song. He could hardly believe it, she was dancing while he lay there in this ludicrous position with his pants down and his hairy bottom exposed.

What could have been a serious, melodramatic situation was being transformed. Jane was a nurse healer. It was not that she intended mockery or to make light of Sam's situation, it was just that it was natural for her to be cheerful. Jane was one of those people who without conscious awareness or practice just seemed to have a knack for balancing a situation. In Sam's case she naturally eased a possibly tense situation by music and movement, all done spontaneously and without premeditation. It was just her style.

In Radiology

"Take it easy now as you lay down, the table may feel hard." Beth lowered her unusually heavy upper torso onto the narrow, sheet-covered x-ray table. Automatically, she pulled up her knees to protect her abdomen and lessen the knife-sharp pain that seemed to cut through her back and down to the groin. "Hey now you are doing great. You know I had five kidney stones myself," said the x-ray technician. "The first one was a lulu, mostly I think because I was scared and didn't know what was happening to me. Then they became kind of like anniversary presents, I got one every year for the next five years."

The large, round-bellied man laughed as he moved around the room positioning the equipment and stacking the film in preparation for picture taking. Beth was about to undergo a intravenous pyelogram, and had it not been for this large, jovial, garrulous man bouncing around his own, well-known territory, she might have been panicked. However, despite her pain, she was amused and distracted. Also, he had survived five diagnosed stones, and they were not even sure if she had one yet. "Yeah," he continued "these stones can be a pain, but what the heck, everyone's gotta have some pain in life. Maybe ours is just gonna be kidney stones."

His homespun philosophy appealed to Beth as she relaxed on the metal table and said in French to herself, "C'est la vie, la vie." What will be, will be. The procedure was rapidly completed, and in time, as is the usual case, she was as good as new. Here again is one more instance where the nurse healer has the opportunity to perform joyful service through an everyday procedure. Each time this occurs both the client and the nurse are empowered.

A Joyful Disposition

Mother Teresa, a Albanian Catholic nun, is renown for initiating an order of caregivers who minister to the terminally ill in hospices in India and Nepal. The criteria for selection to serve in her order is not the same as one would find in health-care agencies in developed countries. The primary quality she seeks for her workers is a joyful disposition. The belief is that joyful service empowers. This is true no matter if the service is to assist one in healing and growth or to assist them in the transition process from living to dying. Mother Teresa is one of many who have recognized that a joyful disposition is one of the basic ingredients to becoming an effective healer.

Cultivating A Joyful Disposition

What if a happy disposition does not come naturally; can it be cultivated? In many instances the answer is yes. Most of us are inclined to repeat behavior that has been rewarded. This is as true in joyful service as in any other endeavor. The value in cultivating this attitude is that not only does the recipient of the service feel better when in contact with the server, but the server also reaps rewards. Contrast the personal joy of Jane as she momentarily looses herself in singing and dancing to another caregiver who would react to the same situation by begrudging her time and the fact she had to be at work at all. Individuals like this would more than likely project their own personal dissatisfaction not only onto the other individual but also into their entire work environment.

Healer Reflections

Can I identify instances in which I have responded with a joyful disposition to an unpleasant task? Do I believe I was in some way empowered because of it?

Can I think of a time I felt empowered when someone helped me? Did they have a joyful disposition?

Chapter 9

Caring for Others as an Extension of the Self

*"No stranger to trouble myself,
I am learning to care for the unhappy."*

Virgil (70–19 B.C.)

Empowering Yourself

How would you like to be cared for if you were ill?

Try to identify with the nurse in the first story as you put yourself in the position of caring for someone else.

Allow yourself to experience the suffering of another as if it were your own.

Think about the interconnectedness of all things in the universe and relate that knowledge to the interconnectedness of each human being.

CARING

The nursing literature is replete with new material on caring. Jean Watson (1988), Patricia Benner, and Judith Wrubel (1989) are among those who popularized the term in nursing. Milton Mayeroff (1972) may have begun the movement when he listed and defined eight major ingredients for caring which are as follows:

1. **Knowledge.** In caring we need to know who the other is, what the needs are, and what will help. We need to know about ourselves, our strengths and limitations. Some things we will know cognitively, others intuitively.

2. **Alternating rhythms.** We move between past experiences and the present situation, between narrow and wide frameworks, between attention to detail and attention to the whole. Both are necessary and both are part of caring.

3. **Patience.** It is not that we wait passively for something to happen, it is that we give it our attention while allowing the person to go at their own pace.

4. **Honesty.** This is a positive, often active, confrontation between ourselves and the other. We need to see the other as they are, not as we would like them to be.

5. **Trust.** This involves the appreciation of the other. Sometimes we care too much and overprotect and do not trust that the other can coparticipate. By trusting we have confidence in our ability to help.

6. **Humility.** Humility to see others as existing for themselves, not simply to satisfy our needs. We treat each person and each situation as unique and relate with humility to each event.

7. **Hope.** Hope is not wishful thinking, but an expression of the fullness of the present. The process of caring is possible because hope is always present.

8. **Courage.** When caring we go into the unknown. Courage makes risk taking possible, but courage is not blind. It is informed by knowledge of the past and the present and by trust in our own and the other's ability to grow.

Canadian nurse-philosopher M. Simone Roach (1987) established the "Five C's of Caring" that grew out of her general statement that caring is the human mode of being. She believes that caring is the basic element of being a person, that when we do not care, we lose our "being," and that caring is the way back into "being." Her five C's are as follows:

1. **Compassion:** a way of living born out of an awareness of one's relationship to all living creatures.

2. **Competence:** a state of having the knowledge, judgment, skills, energy, experience, and motivation required to respond adequately to the demands of one's professional responsibilities.

3. **Confidence:** the quality that fosters trusting relationships.

4. **Conscience:** a state of moral awareness; a compass directing one's behavior according to the moral fitness of things.

5. **Commitment:** a complex, affective response characterized by a convergence of one's desires and one's obligations and by a deliberate choice to act in accordance with them.

All of these concepts will be found interwoven with the theory and anecdotes threaded throughout this text. Caring is an integral part of the nurse healer.

Maria's Story

"There now Maria, calm yourself. Look at me now, and take a deep breath. You can control yourself. Look at me as I speak."

"But I miss my mother so much," she sobbed. "It is just so hard being away from her. I miss her so much."

Little, 11-year-old Maria quivered as her weepy, brown eyes met Lisa's. With deep sighs their eyes matched as Lisa continued a firm, steady monologue to Maria about self-control, deep breathing, and maintaining her focus on the sound of her voice. There they were, a first-time camp nurse and a young girl from Mexico City thrust into one another's presence in the middle of a boisterous, bustling summer-camp dining room. Maria felt totally displaced, alienated from her own reality of city life and her native tongue, and abandoned by the mother she adored. When the sounds of the dining room become so loud that they had to gesticulate to one another, Lisa led Maria outside where they could be together without the roar of the crowd.

They crouched down on a huge, granite rock outside. The roar of voices just inside the screens blended into background noise as they lowered themselves to comfort and naturally fell into a cozy position. They cuddled together and picked up the conversation where they left off.

As Maria's eyes filled and spilled over again, she placed her right hand over her abdomen, "My stomach hurts so much," she wailed. The flood of tears matched the pain in her middle as she doubled over.

"I know it hurts," Lisa replied. Little Maria had a stomach ulcer and was on a specific regimen for treatment and control of symptoms. "Maria, do you notice how it hurts more when you cry?"

"Yes," she sobbed, burying her face in her knees simulating a fetal position.

"Maria, I believe your heart and your stomach are connected. When your heart is sad and unhappy, your stomach hurts. What do you think about that?"

"Yes, you are right, my heart is sad."

"Maria, if you understand the connection, then we must find a way to help you have a happy heart."

"How can I be happy when I am so sad? I miss my mother so much. Why does she send me here when I am so unhappy?"

This was not Maria's first summer at camp. She had come the year before and was tearful much of the time then too, but was in satisfactory health. She declared she had told her mother she did not want to return this year. The situation at home, however, was perceived from a different perspective by her mother. Maria's parents were divorced before camp last year, the father left home, and the mother worked outside of the home. The city was hot and smog-filled during the long summer. There was little or nothing for young Maria, an only child, to do to occupy the summer vacation months. Also their relatives from the area came to this same camp and thrived in the woodsy out-of-doors.

"Maria, let us talk about ways for you to have a happy heart. I think we both agree that is what is important and that is what will make your stomach better."

"But, I miss my mother; I love her so much."

"What a lucky mother you have to have such a sweet little girl to love her as much as you do."

"I do love her so much, but I don't think she loves me. How could she love me and send me away to this forest when I did not want to come?"

Lisa gulped, her heart went out to this small, miserable child. She was literally sobbing her heart out, a very unhealthy state, particularly for someone with stomach ulcers. Lisa looked at her and saw a part of herself reflected back. Her own inner child, her own little-girl self related to this child who had arrived without any warning into her adult lap and adult mind.

"Maria, your mother is wiser than you suspect. When she tells you she has your best interests at heart, you must believe her. There are many important lessons to learn in this life, and your mother is aware of things you do not yet know." Her small face was intent on Lisa's. Her young mind wondered if she could help her. Could this new person quiet her deep, unrelenting misery? Lisa took a deep breath, snuggled Maria close to her and continued.

"Maria, in this life people you love come and go. Sometimes you love someone so much, and that someone, for one reason or another, finds they must go away. If that person is the only one we love, then our heart can be broken by their absence. It can be a very sorrowful thing, and you can suffer greatly. That, Maria, is what is happening to you now. I understand your pain for I have experienced it myself."

Lisa told her the story about when she was a camper her age and about her own homesickness. As she spoke, she became the little girl she had been, and it was through these moments and this medium of dialogue and storytelling that they completely connected. Lisa became an actual extension of Maria, and Lisa saw Maria as an extension of herself.

Lisa continued, "Maria, what is important for you to do is to begin to love other people. You cannot go home now and your mother is not here, but other people are here. Do you think you can learn to love other people? Can you love me?"

"Oh yes," she fervently declared, "I do love you, but I miss my mother."

"Of course you miss her, but what is important now is to put your thoughts of her into a special safe place, maybe a small, magical locket that you can wear around you neck. Save and treasure your thoughts and memories, but store them in safekeeping for the next few weeks. Now is the time, and here is the place to learn new skills. To have a happy heart you must learn to love other people. Know that I love you."

"And I love you," she said precisely as the hoard of girls just dismissed from the dining hall came stampeding out. Maria smiled and Lisa gave her a wink as her friends scooped her up to take her off for evening games.

"See you later," Maria said as she linked arms with two other girls and Lisa walked away. Later, Lisa met with the camp director relaying the story and developing a plan to create a mother-surrogate relationship between Maria and Wanda, an older, motherly, senior counselor. Together they would help Maria learn to love others, to curtail the allegorical bleeding of her heart, and to release her pain. They would teach her to heal both her heart and her gut.

Observations

There are many parts to an individual psyche. The mature grown-up incorporates the child within, the adult, and the parent. These correlate with the id, ego, and superego theory of mid–twentieth century psychology. A person may not actually be a parent but integrates aspects of the critical and/or supportive parent into the judgmental aspect of the mature psyche. Likewise, even though the physical child has developed to adulthood, the psychological aspects of the playful and/or hurt child remain in the grown-up. Consequently, an adult working with a child still has their own psychological child within and can pull forth those aspects of themselves to more quickly and easily relate to the child.

In Maria's case Lisa extended her own inner child to Maria in order that Maria sense comprehension and understanding of her plight. Because of Lisa's consciousness sending Maria felt the connection, the bridge building between them. Because Maria knew she carried a similar hurt to what Lisa had experienced, she could relate to her.

To become a healer in the fullest sense one must experience the trials of many of life's challenges. To feel another's suffering it is beneficial for the healer to have some sense of the sorrow of the other. To comprehend the suffering of loss, of sickness, and of sorrow the healer must have some of their own. Through Lisa's extension to this child, she established their interconnectedness and took on her sorrow. By this means Lisa helped her, and by doing so once again experienced the interconnectedness of all matter, of mind and spirit.

Healer Reflections

Do I feel an interconnectedness with the staff and clients with whom I work?

Do I have the capacity to feel the depths of another's emotions as if they were my own?

In what ways can I begin to care for others as if they were an extension of myself?

REFERENCES

Benner, P. & Wrubel, J. *The primacy of caring.* Menlo Park, Calif.: Addison-Wesley Publishing, 1989.

Mayeroff, M. *On caring.* New York: Harper & Row, 1972.

Roach, M. S. *The human act of caring.* Ottawa: Canadian Hospital Association, 1987.

Tschudin, V. *Ethics in nursing: The caring relationship.* Oxford, England: Butterworth-Heinemann Ltd., 1992.

Watson, J. *Nursing: Human science and human care.* New York: National League for Nursing, 1988.

Chapter 10

A Sense of Purpose

"Our whole duty may be to clarify and increase what we are, to make our consciousness a finer quality."

Florida Scott-Maxwell

Empowering Yourself

Consider your purpose in being a nurse?

Observe how people with a sense of purpose will make any situation work.

Identify how having a sense of purpose affects cancer survivors.

PURPOSE

Purpose involves the conscious direction and flow of a person's inner visions toward achieving a stated potential. Nurses are accustomed to meeting goals and objectives. Purpose, while applicable to these finite ends, implies direction at a broader or higher level. A nurse who works with purpose superimposes the guiding principle of health and healing onto all other clinical goals and objectives.

COMING ALIVE WITH MEANING AND PURPOSE

One of the major plights of many in the modern world is their sense of purposelessness, ennui, boredom, and apathy. On the other hand, most nurse healers have embarked on their own self-healing and crossed the river of ennui and apathy. In so doing they emerge with clear and definite purpose. Nurse healers are people who make a difference. What kind of people become all they can be, what kind of people become healers? Can everyone regardless of station in life have a sense of purpose?

People with exceptional ability exist at every level, even the most modest levels of every organization, and in every walk of life. People in the process of becoming begin in every type of job. I recall a unique person I was privileged to observe many years ago. I was a student and he was an elevator operator. He was a man who to others may have seemed totally trapped but whose mission allowed him to succeed in a job that condemned others to a life of utter boredom.

Marvin and the Elevator

One wintry evening coming back from the library I entered the tower residence hall. All the automatic elevators were shut down for the night. The remaining, old, manual elevator was manned by Marvin. As I approached the portal, I heard music. I looked up and could not believe what I saw—Marvin was dancing in the elevator. He gave me a broad smile and, moving in time with the music, eased the doors shut. This scene was quite a contrast from the staid library setting I had just left. Being a student not only of nursing, but also of life, I ask Marvin a standard, research question, "what are you doing?" He replied, "I'm having a party." I replied with a follow-up, "where are the rest of the people?" He said, "They're not invited."

I thought, "This guy is either crazy or he is going to teach me something." I didn't pursue it further then, but I made a mental note to follow up on it. A month later, I did. It was during the middle of the day, the other elevators were down, and there he was dancing in the elevator, the music still playing. When I asked what he was doing, he once again said he was having a party.

At that point I told him that I was interested in people's motivations and that I would like to hear his story. So I asked, "What keeps you going? Why do you always seem so happy? Do you have some sort of mission?"

He replied, "You want to know my mission? Well, I'm going to be a dancer someday. With what they pay in this job, I can't afford dance lessons. So I have the same two choices every other operator has. I can let my dream die, or I can dance in the elevator."

Now here is what I assessed as the key issue. There were 16 other people just like him, with the same job, in this building complex. They had the same work setting but reacted differently to the same stimuli. Most of the people in Marvin's position or similar situations react to their jobs by saying, "My plight is miserable. My supervisor won't let me make any changes. The organization is rotten. My parents stymied me. The school system ruined me." Yet here, in an elevator cage, one person managed to see a different world and a different set of possibilities.

What he was saying to me was, "I can let my dream die or I can make it work anyway." People with a purpose are those who will make any situation work, while everybody else is complaining or talking about their obstacles. The men and women who founded this country, the immigrants who came and then settled the frontiers, made it work anyway. No matter what you want, if you want it badly enough, and if you apply your skills consistently enough, you'll make it work anyway.

People want to be part of the best; they want to make a contribution. When you ask people what is the number one hindrance to their performance, many of them say, "I don't know what this place stands for, I don't know what they want from me, or I don't know what I want to do with my life." What would happen if we did that in nursing or in any other significant endeavor? Thus my focus is on the basic question: What is the significance of mission and purpose?

CANCER SURVIVORS

All of us are interested in cancer survivors. These are people who mystify health professionals. Usually their doctors label them as spontaneous remissions. When you study this issue, you quickly realize that spontaneous remission is a medical euphemism for "we don't know what happened." When you talk to such patients, ask them, "What did you do to survive? Did you do anything that the rest of us can learn from?" You may discover that cancer survivors use the same skills as Marvin in the elevator, as the great leaders in business, or as the great scientists and artists.

What they consistently say is, "I draw on resources I never knew I had. I draw on talents I never knew were there. I am tougher than I thought." One man, a nationally known actor, said, "What I did in that hospital, to stay alive, was the hardest thing I ever did, much harder than my performances on stage. It was my peak performance."

When you speak to these people about their jobs, ask them, "What did you do that the rest of us could learn from?" Ask them, "If you had only one hour to live, what would be the most important thing to you? What would you think about during your last hour on Earth?" It turns out they will only talk about two things. They talk about the people they love and that they want more time to love more, and they talk about work. They are particularly proud of work that makes an impact. Not one of those people would ever say, with an hour left to live, "I would think of my bank account." Nobody mentions possessions of any kind. They talk about love and work, which I believe is the starting point for each of our own missions. What work are you proud of, and who are you doing it for? Who do you care about? These are the important questions to ask. As we become healers of both self and others, these are the questions we need to repeatedly ask. It is through finding meaning in our work and purpose in our life that we are most likely to experience fulfillment.

CRISIS IN MEANING AND VALUES

For many people there is a crisis in meaning and values. No need is so compelling as the need we all feel for our lives to make sense, to have meaning. We will tolerate almost any degree of austerity or risk in this indomitable quest for meaning and purpose. After the "great debunking" of religion by reductionists and science and with the discovery that economic production, consumption, and even technological achievement are unfulfilling, many in modern society feel a vacuum in the area of basic values and central meaning.

The incompleteness of science and its inability to deal with the whole human experience is being challenged by a rapidly developing interest in philosophical and religious outlooks, a renaissance in Western mysticism, and a vast array of explorations of the world of inner experience—from yoga and meditative disciplines to confrontation therapies and psychedelic drug experiences. Within science a similar opening of interests is occurring, manifesting in humanistic and transpersonal psychology, exploration of altered states of consciousness, and other areas. There are multifold signs of a respiritualization of Western society, with emphasis on self-realization, transcendental meaning, and inner growth leading to wisdom and compassion.

THE IMPORTANCE OF ATTITUDE

Perhaps the single most important category of attributes of a healer is attitude, for it is from attitudes that behaviors flow. Healing behaviors are manifest by the person who has developed the attitudes delineated in the four chapters in this section. In Part V we will identify and explore how these attitudes are manifest in healing behaviors.

Healer Reflections

What is the mission in my life?

Can I identify personal weaknesses that I can channel into creative strengths?

In what ways does Marvin reflect attitudes that I would like to foster?

Of what work am I proud and for whom am I doing it?

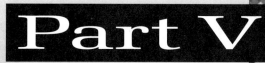

Part V

Cultivating

Healing

Behaviors

Chapter

Outward Expressions
of the Inner Light

*Nursing is no more and no less than the professionalization
of the human capacity to care through the acquisition and
application of the knowledge, attitudes, and skills appropriate to nursing's prescribed roles.*

Sister Simone M. Roach

Empowering Yourself

Note how the healers in this chapter's stories think, speak,
and act from their center—from a place of authenticity.

Identify how and why forgiveness works to calm and balance a healer's inner being.

Consider the different kinds of expressions of healing.

LIVING FROM A PLACE OF AUTHENTICITY

All of us at some time or another wrestle with questions of authenticity. Are we who we say we are? Do our actions represent what we profess to believe, or is some nature of our being hypocritical? Is our behavior contradictory to professed beliefs? Do we walk the path of authenticity, or is there subtle or even frank ambiguity between our attitudes and our behaviors?

To be an effective healer one must be authentic. In the mystical, metaphoric realm where there is still conjecture about how actual healing occurs, one thing is certain; one who would be a healer must be genuine. Within this illusive realm there is no room for self-serving or charlatan activities. Only those with genuine intent become healers.

Those who live from a place of authenticity generally exhibit three universal qualities that are inherent in the healing process. The qualities expressed through the healing behaviors are forgiveness, love, and compassion.

FORGIVENESS

Most people carry grudges, and what are grudges but unforgiven issues, mostly silenced and/or repressed, but still operant in our lives. Grudges are derived from emotional hurts that have not been healed but instead have shifted from a conscious initial hurt into mostly subconscious chronic wounds. Perhaps one of the most dramatic and powerful aspects of our humanness is how we continue to carry the burden of our hurts, rejections, criticisms, and disappointments, ostensibly inflicted on us by others. How often do you hear statements such as . . . "my mother was so cruel, and I have had to suffer the consequences ever since," or "I can never trust another man again after what he did to me," or "watch out, even your best friend may betray you." These and many similar variations are typical in the contemporary world, and they all smack of the need to forgive.

A memorable book written during the 1970s broaches this subject. Laura Huxley wrote a series of essays published under the title of the lead essay, *You Are Not the Target*. In this classic work she describes how often we "react" when people snap at us or seem rude and inconsiderate. When we have made a genuine effort to be helpful or kind or have accidentally done something and evoked a hostile reaction, what is important for us to remember is that in most cases we are not at fault but are simply a target for another's pent-up frustrations. This psychological system is analogous to the Oriental physical defense system of akido in which you deflect onslaught blows instead of combating them as you would in the defense system of karate. Rather than "reacting" back, the preferable action is to deflect the verbal assault by letting it bypass our stored memory bank. If we "take it on," we accept someone else's unresolved and chaotic issues. Both verbally and physically we can learn to deflect rather than combat assaults.

To carry this concept a step further let us consider an additional step, the act of forgiveness. There is much deliberate and unintentional ill will in the world, and likewise there is much holding and harboring of it. When we understand the need for and practice forgiveness, we will each do a part in releasing some of the "held" anger and resentment so prevalent in the world today. If each of us practiced forgiveness and release in our own daily practice, the mass holding of negative energies might shift.

If we agree in theory that forgiveness is a laudable goal, then where and how do we begin? Remember the old adage, "charity begins at home." Forgiveness, similar to charity and other virtues, probably works best when we start with the basics, when we begin at home.

Carol's Story

Many women go to self-growth or empowerment workshops. Carol was one. She is memorable because of her remarkable story of forgiveness. Carol and her group were seated in a semicircle at the base of a huge, stone fireplace on the Saturday night of a woman's wellness weekend workshop. Each participant took a turn at telling a story of a primary empowering event in their life. Carol chose to tell the story of her family. She began by telling her group about her mother, Sally.

It seems Sally's mother (Carol's grandmother) locked her in dark closets, beat her with a hairbrush, and eventually when she was older actually tried to compete with Carol for the men in her life. In early adulthood Sally banned her mother from her life and swore she would never speak to her again. She remarried and soon thereafter had a baby whom she named Carol. Shortly following the birth of her child, her husband left her for another woman. Poor, embittered, and alone, Sally struggled for survival. She took a full-time day job and part-time evening and night work. She found a family in a neighboring town whom she paid to keep her baby. She was only able to visit one

Sunday a month when she was off work. Sally struggled to make ends meet. When Carol was old enough to ask questions about her father and her grandmother, she was told that they were no good and that they were better off without them.

Throughout Carol's young life she got the idea that men were wicked and old women were meddlesome. The message she learned was that to survive you have to work hard, be wary of men, and be very certain about who you trust. Although Sally's gentle child loved her mother, she also loved her grandmother. As Carol matured to womanhood, she saw the furrows of anger and resentment crease her mother's tired face. Through independent counseling and group therapy she learned about the concept of forgiveness. Carol was determined to integrate this practice in her daily life. The first person she consciously chose to forgive was her own mother, Sally. Carol had grown up hearing that men were cruel and not to be trusted. She was often reminded that her father had abandoned her. It was understandable then that Carol herself had difficulty trusting men. Also she had been taught that one's own mother could be meddlesome, and actually Sally was now becoming an annoyance to Carol. It was during therapy that Carol recognized that she was taking on similar characteristics to her mother. She began to understand the vicious cycle that had been born and firmly resolved to break the cycle with her generation. Carol committed to making operant the phenomenon of forgiveness in her life. She saw where she must begin. Forgiveness, she realized begins at home.

How did she operationalize the concept? Carol knew that her mother could never accept the fact that maybe she had been wrong about men or about her own mother. Consequently she did not endeavor to change her mother's actions or belief patterns. The person she worked on was herself. She diligently worked to create a mental image of her mother as a young and helpless girl who had no doubt been molded by trauma that swept through her developmental years. Sally had, after all, done the best possible job she could have done with the circumstances she faced and the insight she had. Carol completely forgave her mother, although not orally or in any physically demonstrative fashion that Sally was ever aware of. Carol forgave Sally in her heart. Because of this she softened to her mother, now elderly, and on whatever occasions were appropriate she found ways to honor her. In time the two women became close, and there seemed to be a physical change in Sally. She lived alone in a city apartment, and on the occasions of Carol's visits they would stroll the city streets and visit old haunts from the past. They would link arms, and because of Carol's consistent mental attitude of forgiveness, both of the past and of occasional current irritants, they could also link hearts. Carol became a master of forgiveness in all areas of her life. She did so because she began with the most complex and yet most important place, she began and achieved mastery at home. From this point Carol projected the ingrained mental behavior of forgiveness into all situations and with people she encountered in her daily life.

Table 11-1
Twelve Ways to Forgiveness

1. At first, pray for just the WILLINGNESS to forgive!

2. Later, pray for the POWER to forgive!

3. Pray for the HEALING of that person's deep inner pain that must have caused that person to hurt you.

4. Visualize that person as a "CHILD OF GOD." Then also visualize yourself as another "child of God."

5. Make sure our own house is clean; as we tend to despise in others the qualities we despise in ourselves.

6. Make sure that we have made amends to ALL other persons we have harmed—whether we feel they deserve these amends or not!

7. Make a LIST of the other person's GOOD qualities, but do NOT list the bad qualities.

8. Make a habit of SAYING SOMETHING GOOD about this person to another person—even if you have to exaggerate.

9. SEND AWAY thoughts of resentment as soon as they occur, and do not chew them over like a cow chews its cud.

10. Make yourself DO A FAVOR for the other person, without letting the source be known.

11. Assume that your forgiveness, whether expressed or not, WILL NOT CHANGE the other person or the attitude toward you; it will ONLY change you!

12. GIVE THANKS to God for the progress, however small, that you have made in forgiveness and for the spiritual peace it brings!

Anonymous

LOVE

The Greeks were the first in the Western tradition to systematize and describe love. The categories they delineated were eros, agape, and phileo. Eros is a possessive desire or love. It is the driving force for absolute good, therefore the motive underling education, fine arts, and philosophy. Agape is akin to sacrificial, protective, brotherly love. Philia pertains to the drive for community through friendship.

It is possible through each type of love for healing to occur. When people join in eros or romantic love, the components of passion, intimacy, and commitment can and often do serve as a bridge for individual support and transformation.

In recent years there has been much discussion about two seemingly contradictory concepts: altruism and enlightened selfishness. If you are altruistic, can you also be selfish? If you are selfish, can you become a healer? Can both qualities coexist in one person?

In the 1950s and 1960s Ayn Rand wrote a group of popular novels in which the heroes and heroines always emerged from the masses and saved the populace, not because they were altruistic, but to the contrary, because of enlightened self-interest. The two concepts of heroism and selfishness almost seem incompatible, yet on close analysis we see that those who conscientiously develop and know "self" first are less likely to get sidetracked by ego traps and other self-justifying, subconscious behaviors.

Twenty years later, in the 1980s, more books about enlightened selfishness appeared and quickly became best-sellers. Most of these books are targeted to women with titles such as *Men Who Can't Love* and *Women Who Love Too Much.*

The message in these books is that people often flounder in sexual love relationships because they have not sufficiently developed the self. Love relationships demand that each individual be psychologically strong to enter such a partnership. The chances of longevity with one strong and one weak partner is remote. Therefore, enlightened selfishness comes first. This means take care of your own stuff before you enter into relationships with significant others. Otherwise, you will end up using the stock psychological defense mechanisms of denial, projection, and rationalization to justify your own unenlightened perspective. The result is often a lose-lose situation with both partners being hurt and disempowered. If this has happened to you,

you can, with sufficient insight, turn the situation into a win-win situation by beginning to work on and learn to love and honor your own self first.

Table 11-2
Love is ...

Slow to suspect
>*–quick to trust.*

Slow to condemn
>*–quick to justify.*

Slow to offend
>*-quick to defend.*

Slow to expose
>*–quick to shield.*

Slow to reprimand
>*–quick to forbear.*

Slow to belittle
>*–quick to appreciate.*

Slow to demand
>*–quick to give.*

Slow to provoke
>*–quick to conciliate.*

Slow to hinder
>*–quick to help.*

Slow to resent
>*–quick to forgive.*

>*Love will find a way!*

Anonymous

Tough Love

Operating from a loving perspective is not always light, soft, and easy. The nurses in the following story depict a quality of "tough love," or love that comes with fortitude and conviction.

Old Mabel Brown

"Open up, Mother. I'm going to put your teeth back in now." Mabel's daughter, Dawn, had been vigorously scrubbing Mabel's false teeth.

She walked back from the sink and forced Mabel's mouth open to reinsert her dentures. "Now then, Mother, you look just fine." Mabel was clean, brushed, and dressed. "All right, Mother, you rest now while I go get your nurse to give your medications."

Dawn made her way down the hall to the nurse's station on Unit Two. "Nurse, my mother is ready for her medications now."

"Hello, Dawn, how are you today?" the charge nurse asked.

"Okay, I suppose. I'll be okay as long as Mother is all right."

"Say Dawn, one of our nurse specialists here at Havenside has asked me to let her know the next time you were in so she can come and talk to you."

"Why, what about?" Dawn retorted. "I thought everything was just fine."

"Well, yes, everything is fine, it is just that she wants to talk to you."

"Why would I need to talk to a nurse specialist?"

"Let her tell you why herself. I will call her and tell her you are here. Until she arrives, I will go back to your mother's room with you and give your mother her medications."

Dawn stood at the counter at Unit Two as the nurse made her call and then walked to the medication room to draw up Mabel's drugs. Both to the left and to the right of the central station Dawn's gaze lit on the rows of old people in wheelchairs. Some chatted with one another, but most stared with unseeing vision at nothing in particular.

"Okay, Dawn, let's go down to your mother's room. I have her medication prepared." The nurse carried a tray with a 50-ml Toomey syringe filled with colored liquid and another filled with water.

They arrived at Mabel's bedside. "Hello, Mother, here is the nurse to give your medications." The nurse looked down at Mabel. Her position had not altered since she turned her two hours previously. She remained as she had been, contracted, contorted, unresponsive, and mute. The nurse advanced to Mabel's feeding tube, clamped the tube, and inserted the Toomey syringe into the G-button site. Swiftly she pushed the plunger, then switched syringes, and flushed the tube with water before reconnecting the liquid feeding.

"Turning to Dawn the nurse said, "Now I am going to send in the nurse's aide to clean and turn your mother. She has been incontinent again. Why don't you come down to the nurses' station with me. The clinical specialist should be along soon, and you can talk with her in our conference room." Compliantly, Dawn moved to follow the nurse.

"See you later, Mother."

Helen, the clinical nurse specialist was standing at the nurses' station when Dawn and the staff nurse arrived. "Hello, Dawn, I have been looking forward to meeting you. Let's go into the conference room and sit down."

Once seated, Helen continued. "You must wonder why I want to talk to you?"

"Yes, I do."

"As the staff nurse told you, I am a consultant here at Havenside. Officially I am a nurse thanatologist. But, before you ask, let me explain what that means. What I do is work with clients and their families to assist them in the dying process."

"I don't see what that has to do with me."

"Well, Dawn, that is actually part of the reason we are meeting now. You see the team that cares for your mother has observed that you do not seem to acknowledge that she is terminally ill. There seems to be some discrepancy between her deteriorating condition and your acceptance of it. Do you understand what I am saying?

Dawn's lower lip quivered. "Mom could go on a long time, you know."

"Do you really think so?"

"Well, doctors and scientists are always coming up with cures."

"That's true, but let's examine the facts in your mother's case. Mabel is 87 years old. She has been crippled with arthritis for over 20 years and had a debilitating stroke four years ago. She has not recognized anyone or spoken since that time."

"Why are you telling me this? Don't you think I know. After all, it has been me who has cared for Mother all these years."

"Of course you have, and that is laudable. I bring this up now because I think it may be time for you to reexamine the quality of your mother's life, not solely the quantity of years she survives. It also may be time for you to reflect on what her passing means to you. You know some people cling to life to the extent that they begin to deny or at least block the fact that death is inevitable. When blocking becomes a pattern, it is difficult to recognize."

"Dawn, you may not know this, but all of us are actually dying and being reborn all the time. We are composed of billions of cells. Thousands of cells slough off and new ones are reformed on a daily basis, which means we are dying and being reborn on a continual basis. In our circulatory system red blood cells are replaced every 120 days, all our skin cells are replaced every four weeks, and bone cells are replaced every four days. In fact, every five years we have an entirely new body."

"What this means, Dawn, is that physical life is a continual renewal process. Your mother's spiritual life may be more difficult to ascertain, but consider this. If the body dissipates and rebuilds, then perhaps so too does the spirit. Is it possible that much of your mother's spirit has already left her and she is simply awaiting your release of her physical form? I raise these questions to you, Dawn, because your mother's care team has recognized the holding-on process that is consuming so much of your life's energy. What I am trying to do, Dawn, is help you refocus on what death means to you. Once you do that, I think it will be easier for you to talk with us about allowing your mother her final release."

"Do you recall your mother's wishes on her living will prior to her stoke? She asked for no heroics, yet for the past two years she has been sustained on internal tube feedings. I do not mean to be harsh, Dawn, but I think it is time for you to consider your mother's requests and why we have been prolonging the inevitable."

"Nurse, this is so difficult for me. I have tried so hard to be a good daughter."

"You have been an excellent daughter, and of course talking about death and dying is difficult. Dawn, I bring this topic up because the staff here cares about you and your mother. It may take a little time for you to think about the things I have brought up today, but I think it is important. I want you to think about redirecting our approach to your mother's care. Can we meet again in two days to talk some more?"

"Sure, I guess it's time I faced the facts. Thank you for spending time with me."

Observation

These nurses cared enough about Dawn and her mother Mabel to force an unpleasant issue to consciousness and to gently, but effectively, demand that it be acknowledged and dealt with.

Altruism

Altruism, a recognized virtue of doing acts to benefit others, is a concept that has come under scrutiny in recent years. What is in question is the motivation behind the act. Pure altruism, without any ulterior motive by the doer is laudable, but it is the sorting out of hidden motives that is difficult. I raise this issue because people can deceive themselves when doing good works. On the surface it appears both to the unexamined self and to the recipient that acts are performed solely for the benefit of the recipient. In fact, on analysis, unconscious or hidden motivation by the doer may occur.

What this means is that the doer may be seeking some sort of social or psychological remuneration because of the act or acts performed. This is usually at the subconscious level of the doer. The problem with this is that these acts can and often do provoke untoward effects or outcomes rather than the anticipated benefit.

Thus the examined life is the better path. Healers in particular must scrutinize their motivations and actions, and if they become altruistic should do so from the level of basic goodness, not from the place of consciously or subconsciously expecting or anticipating reward.

COMPASSION

Compassion is more than simple kindness or caring. We can care without having compassion. Compassion leads us to go where it hurts, to enter places of pain, to share in brokenness, fear, confusion, and anguish. Compassion challenges us to cry out with those in misery, mourn with those who are lonely, or to weep with those who cry. Compassion means full immersion in the condition of being human.

Barbara's Story

Barbara was in her mid-forties while working at a large hospital in the South. She became divorced many years ago shortly after the birth of her son and had been his sole support for the past 10 years. For the next seven years Barbara was a cheerful and dedicated employee and a committed mother. While they lived in the South, her son Philip attended the local public high school and Barbara did her best to be a good mother. Whenever he brought friends home, she always had milk and cookies, fresh fruit, and plenty of smiles. Following Philip's high school graduation, Barbara and Philip decided to return to their birthplace and moved back home to the Northeast.

At this point they became serious about Philip's education and combed the Northeast for a school that would accept him at his level of preparation and support his future growth. Barbara and his counselors felt that Philip needed a small college where he could have personalized attention. The year Philip was 18 they visited schools in the northeast on all their days off. Philip got a job in a cafeteria and tried to juggle his days off to match his mother's who, despite her higher education, could only find a job as a staff nurse in the community in which they settled. During this first year back in New England, both mother and son saved all their money after meeting basic living expenses. They also finally located an excellent school that would meet Philip's needs. The only problem was that the tuition, fees, books, and room and board totaled $29,000 a year. The college financial advisor examined the family income but stated that Philip was not eligible for financial aid because his father earned a high income. The problem was, however, that the father was estranged from the pair and would not agree to pay anything for college.

Barbara once again in her life "bit the bullet," and taking the plunge, enrolled Philip for the following fall. She had a choice in how to respond, and she did what was needed to empower them both. Now, not only did she have to support herself, but had to net an additional $20,000 annually for Philip's schooling. Philip himself could earn the $9,000 difference. True to her nature Barbara got busy seeking a new job that would earn the necessary income and at the same time launch an independent business, something she had wanted to do her whole life. So, in Barbara's fifty-fifth year and Philip's twentieth, she went back to work and he started college.

Barbara's speciality was gerontology, the care of the elderly. She had been a caring person and a good mother all her life, but her true compassionate nature opened with the new purposeful activity that began with Philip's education.

During Philip's first year at college she opened her new business, CEI, Creative Education Integration. With her advanced degrees and thirty years of nursing experience she was able to offer educational programs to nursing homes to train their off-the-street personnel in how to give humanistic care to the elderly. To support both her week-day business during its formative years and her son's expenses, Barbara was forced to take a second job for additional income. She obtained a job as a staff nurse in a nursing home. This was not a regular position, but to get the pay she required, she agreed to work 12-hour shifts, 7 A.M. to 7 P.M. every Saturday and Sunday for 1 year. She would be given two weekends off during the 12-month period.

Barbara did have clinical experience and certainly knew the theory, but what she encountered and the feelings evoked in her in this setting were not what she had expected. On her first weekend she came to the job feeling energetic and enthusiastic; she was ready to work. However, because she was an RN, the director assigned her the more difficult patients. And who were they? Almost without exception everyone of them was withered, frail, helpless, cranky, incontinent, deaf, blind, and terminally ill. It was Barbara's assignment to bathe, feed, medicate, and turn and position them, treat their bedsores, and last, but not least, give them nurturing. Her first weekend was exhausting. Even though she had taught and even directed a school of nursing, she was not prepared for the reality shock of elder care in contemporary American nursing homes. What she encountered jolted her to the core. Here within the confines of physically isolated, long-term care facilities were the rejected beings of our own technological health care revolution. Mere physical shells of forgotten grandmothers and grandfathers lay curled in embryonic positions. They were thin-skinned skeletons of organisms only remnant of what once had been. They were beings whose spirits were crushed as calloused personnel carelessly tossed and bumped them about or painted their withered faces with bright lipstick and rouge and then laughed at their helplessness while they sat imprisoned, strapped in, one after another in a row of wheelchairs facing a meaningless series of incomprehensible color flashes on a television screen.

Occasionally a plea of, "Oh God, please help me," emanated from a toothless mouth, interrupting the incomprehensible stream of words flowing from the television. Other times a yellow puddle of fluid would appear on the floor from a diaper or Chux pad overflow from one of the few who had not yet had a permanent, indwelling, urinary-catheter insertion.

Barbara did the best she could working her 12-hour weekend shifts. She fed, tended, and observed an isolated, abandoned segment of the population, outcast because of a society who does not know how to deal with it.

Compassion—what does it mean? At a recent conference one of the speakers likened this term to the African song "Kumbyya" or "come by with passion." Faithfully, each weekend for 50 consecutive weeks Barbara and others like her left the outside world and came to be with elders. They did so with passion: passion for caring, passion for feeling. Barbara felt a tremendous empathy for these discarded elders, often comparing them to how her own parents might be soon, and she hoped they would receive similar compassionate care as she gave here.

The other thing that happened with Barbara because of her tenure at this nursing home was her developing an awareness of and arriving at a conclusion in favor of the controversial issue of euthanasia, or "mercy killing." During her care she witnessed that many of these beings had moved beyond the state of ordinary, redemptive suffering and, being mere shadows of their former self, were actually almost punished because they had the unfortunate fate of living beyond their normal life span. This is true in most cases because of technological interventions for which they had not asked. Old grandmothers and grandfathers lingered with feeding tubes taped to their noses and catheters between their legs.

Barbara participated mechanically as she was instructed to insert needles into the backs of old hands with tissue-thin skin for the purpose of allowing the drip of antibiotic liquids into sclerotic veins to further prolong their helpless life.

Day after day, week after week, Barbara went there with passion. She always did her best, but she increasingly asked why. Why are we prolonging the life of these souls who are so frail, so sick, so terminal?

At the end of a year's time Philip had successfully completed his first year of college, and Barbara had had her heart opened by witnessing suffering she had not known before. Because of her compassion for their plight she learned about euthanasic practices in the Netherlands and about the Hemlock Society in California. She discovered a group of compassionate consumers sincerely concerned about the issues and practice of humanistic death and dying and learned about living wills and her legal rights to prevent the prolongation of her own life.

Healer Reflections

Do I practice my nursing skills from a place of authenticity?

Who do I need to forgive?

Do I consider "tough love" a form of loving expression?

Am I aware that altruism has a shadow side. Are my altruistic expressions genuine?

In what ways do I express compassion in my everyday practice?

Chapter 12

Characteristic Behaviors

Character is a natural power like light and heat and all nature cooperates with it.

Ralph Waldo Emerson (1803–1882)

Empowering Yourself

Identify ways you can become more fully present as you interact with clients.

Consider your listening skills as you read the story about Betty Barns.

Acknowledge that empathy is a primary concept employed by nurse healers.

Note that attention to detail is a necessary part of delivering quality client care when the overall purpose is healing.

BEING FULLY PRESENT

Nurse healers use all their senses to be completely present during the moments of successful healing encounters. Being fully present includes developing listening skills, attending to detail, and learning the art of empathy.

Trauma Healing: Tommy's Story

"Help, somebody help us, he's bleeding." Not unaccustomed to trauma, Robin, a nurse at the local hospital, tossed down her popcorn and quickly entered the roller-skating rink. Three swift skate strokes later she arrived at Tommy's side, and sure enough, there was blood gushing from his face. Following a quick physical assessment Robin ascertained that he had no other major injuries except the overt bleeding from his nasopharnyx region.

"Okay Tommy, get up. I'm going to take you over to the bench." Looking directly into his eyes he matched Robin's gaze and followed her authoritative direction. Together, skate to skate, they glided and wobbled their way to the side. Within seconds Robin had him lying on a bench against the wall that encircled the roller-skating rink. Oblivious to anything else she kept her attention fixed on Tommy as she commanded to one of the gapping onlookers, "Get me some ice and paper towels from the concession stand. The rest of you move back so we will have some more room."

"Now breathe deeply and think of something pleasant," Robin said. "I'm going to move my hand for a moment and look into your mouth." As she moved her hand to release the pressure over his mouth, blood gushed from the area of his upper lip. She replaced her hand and said, "Tommy, now I want you to slow your breathing. I have my hand over your mouth, so breath deeply through your nose. Here we go now, in through your nose, pause and now out." After a few more breaths she felt his panic begin to subside. He stopped trembling. "Tommy, you're going to be okay." Just then someone shoved a paper towel encasing some ice into Robin's hand lying on Tommy's shoulder. Without looking up she thanked them and placed the ice pack over Tommy's lip. "Now, let's continue, breathe in deeply and release it, good, that's the idea. Now again." After few more times of this she said, "Tommy, the ice has been on a while now, so I'm going to release my hand, remove the ice and take another look." This time the bleeding had clearly stopped. There was a small laceration on the lip where the tooth had punctured the skin when he fell to the wooden floor. Obviously, there would be no need for emergency care. Realizing the bleeding had stopped, Tommy sat up.

"I feel much better now. Can I have a drink?"

"Good idea," Robin declared as she sent another unknown child to get Tommy a coke. Suddenly the crowd that had hovered around during the excitement had apparently disbursed and returned to skating. Tommy and Robin sat chatting as the coke carrier returned and delivered the drink to the waiting boy.

They sat a few more minutes as he gulped the drink and then said, "Can I skate again now?"

"It's all right with me, but don't you want to call home and tell them about your fall."

"Naw, I feel fine now. I'll tell them when I get home. So with a puffy, red lip and tear-stained cheeks little Tommy, whom Robin had never seen before and would likely never see again, shyly thanked her. Before she could answer, he skated off into rink and became indistinguishable in the crowd from which only minutes ago he had emerged.

Observations

During the healing process healers are rarely distractible. The act of healing requires full presence. Begin fully present is a skill that can be acquired but rarely has to be. That is because during the healing act itself the healer's attention naturally focuses on the act and with the person, which is the nature of healing. During the time Robin was with Tommy she had no cognition of the people surrounding her, how long the healing act took, or the fact the care took place in a setting with an extraordinarily high noise level. This nurse healer's attention was completely focused on the child and the desire to stop the bleeding.

....

The following is a list of ways to increase "being fully present":

- Situate your body so you directly face the person with whom you are working.
- Focus eye contact on the person receiving attention.
- Focus mental thoughts on the immediate event.
- Block distracting motion, words, and sounds from entering your conscious attention.

LISTENING

An essential aspect of communication is effective listening. Active listening includes eye contact, attentive nonverbal behavior, and a genuine effort to be emphathic. Listening of this type prepares the nurse healer to clearly reflect the client's thoughts and feelings so that a genuine understanding both by the client and the nurse will occur.

Betty's Story

"Diane, this is Betty Barnes, could I talk to you for a few minutes?" Diane was busy but knew if Betty were calling, it must be important to her.

"What's up?" Diane said. "It's been a year since I've heard from you. Are you okay?" Betty was one of those numerous people in life whom you get to know and like, but the relationship stays on an acquaintance level rather than developing into a full-fledged friendship only because there is not enough time to devote to fostering a meaningful friendship. She was one of those people Diane liked to keep up with, but did not see or talk to often.

"I've had some hard times lately," Betty replied. "You know I don't talk readily and easily to many people, but I'm having so much trouble and facing some difficult decisions, and I just wondered if you would see me professionally, to counsel me?"

Diane was quick to reply, "Betty, I closed my client-based counseling practice last year and I am no longer doing that, but I will see and talk to you as a friend. Can you come over?"

"I couldn't bother you like that. I'll only come if I can pay you."

"Nonsense, I wouldn't charge you even if I still had my practice." Diane knew she was adjusting to the financial strains of a divorce and was between jobs as well. "Let me get my schedule and let's find a good time for both of us. Okay, how about three o'clock this afternoon?"

"Are you sure? I don't want to impose on you."

"Don't worry, come over then and we'll have tea and talk. See you then." Diane hung up the phone knowing Betty must be in some sort of pain; she was not someone who asked without need. Diane readjusted her afternoon schedule and went back to work.

Promptly at three o'clock Betty arrived. She entered apologetically leaning on a cane and carrying a rubber, air-filled ring encased in a pillowcase. "Come in," Diane greeted and gave her a hug. "Let's go back to my office and sit down." She had already prepared a pot of herbal tea and had it brewing.

"If you don't mind I'd like to stand for a while. I had to sit in the car on the way over here and I can't sit for very long at a time anymore. Mostly I have to lie flat, however, I brought my special cushion along for when I do sit." Diane's mental wheels churned; Betty only lived a 15-minute drive away—she must be in intense pain.

"Okay, come walk down the hall with me while I get the tea tray." Betty hobbled along behind her. "Betty, you are obviously having more physical problems than when I saw you last," Diane said as she launched into the reason for which she had probably come.

Diane had known Betty for about five years, mostly professionally, and had always liked her spunky nature and willingness to try new, innovative approaches. She worked well with people and had many of the attributes of a healer herself. Now at what should be the peak of her life, she was in trouble. At 35 she appeared to be at the ebb of life. Heading back down the hall with the tea tray they entered Diane's cozy office, and after resting the tray and pouring the tea, they sat down. Betty circled the chair, adjusted her cushion, and carefully lowered her tiny frame deftly over the circle of air.

"My back is worse. I'm in pain all the time. I didn't renew my teaching contract last year. None of my colleagues know the severity of my pain. I'm so embarrassed, they think I took the year off to travel. I thought I'd be better by now. It's been 6 months, but I'm no better, and the money is running out. My parents have offered to help, but I so want to be independent." She raced on, with all the pain and misery of 6 months of confinement flowing out, as Diane sat across from her transfixed by the outpouring of suffering. Betty continued, "I've been to the pain clinic, and they have me on some potent analgesics, but full relief is seldom. What I want is your opinion and advice about the options I've delineated." She looked at her watch, "but I don't want to take up too much of your time."

"Betty, relax. I have the time to spend with you now." Settling back she took her first sip of what by then must have been cold tea. She didn't seem to notice.

"I guess the divorce hit me harder than I expected it too. I feel so alone. He took everything, I didn't care. At least I don't have to see him now. I just never expected it. And now all this pain to boot. How could life have been so rosy, and now it's so bleak? But I don't want to get mired down in self-pity, so here are what I see as options. First, what do you think about this Pain and Rehabilitation Center in California. I've heard the doctors there can turn around chronic neurological pain. Is this true?" She thrust a brochure about the clinic into Diane's hand. "Second, since I can't hold a job now, what do you think about taking charity from my family? They have offered to let me move back in with them, but it would make me feel so dependent. What would you do in this case? The other thing I would like to do is study and read, but that seems so lazy, what do you think? Honestly, I feel so weak for not being able to come to terms with these issues by myself, but if you don't mind, I really would value your opinion."

Over the next few minutes Diane responded to her questions and gave her the feedback she requested. Betty affirmed that Diane's opinions matched her own, yet Diane was unsure at the time if she only said that to please her. Diane sensed that the other thing Betty needed and was reticent to ask for was someone to really listen to her. Any sincere listener would have been moved to compassion and been willing to direct her to get the care she so obviously needed. They talked an hour away and then as promptly and politely as she arrived, Betty left.

Diane did not hear from her again for another year when once again, as unexpectedly as the previous year, Betty called. "Hi," she said, "I called to tell you I followed all of your suggestions and I am much better. I went to the Pain Clinic and was able to get long-term relief. I moved in with my parents and have spent the year in seclusion reading and studying. At this point I am about to reenter the outside world, and I wanted you to be the first to know. I simply wanted to thank you for the answers and information you gave me last year. In a way, you saved my life. I shall be eternally grateful." After a few pleasantries we hung up. A few months later Diane saw Betty in the grocery store, still with a cane, but also with a smile and an obvious sense of independence, a trait she prized over many others.

Observations

The desire and ability to listen is one of the behaviors of healers. One never knows when important moments, windows of healing opportunities, will emerge. Through the vehicle of genuine listening healing can be evoked.

Listening Traps

Sometimes even nurse healers become so involved and rushed in trying to accomplish their work we forget some of the essentials of effective listening. Even we can lapse into poor listening skills.

Answer the following list of 10-point questions and rate yourself to check your listening skills. Answer yes, no, or sometimes. If you have a predominance of "yes" or "sometimes" responses, you might consider working on your listening skills.

1. Does your mind tend to wander and think about something else when your client is talking to you?

2. Are you so involved in your own feelings that it is impossible to let go of your own thoughts and really listen to another?

3. Do you mentally tune the other person out to prepare your own response to the issue under discussion?

4. Do you tend to jump ahead of the speaker and reach conclusions before you have heard the speaker out?

5. Do you often think you know what the other person is going to say before he or she has finished saying it?

6. Are you in a hurry to impart your ideas to the conversation or relate your experiences when the other is talking?

7. Do you have a tendency to finish sentences or supply words for the other person?

8. Do you get caught up with insignificant facts and details and miss the emotional tone of the conversation?

9. Do you listen with half your attention tuned toward giving advice, solving the problem, or figuring out what to say to make the other person feel better rather than allowing the person to finish speaking before trying to solve their problem?

10. Do you realize that good listening skills take consistent effort?

EMPATHY

Empathy is the art of communicating to others that we have understood how they are feeling and what makes them feel that way. It is closely related to listening but goes a step beyond.

An Educator's Experience

The group of four health-care professionals approached the bed in the semidarkened room. A frail, elderly woman was lying semiconscious, her withered face turned upward and unseeing eyes gazing into a dimension beyond our huddled group. The lights flickered on as one of the students began to prepare the patient and the site for the demonstration to the other students of how to do a neurological status check. All the attention was focused on the bed as the conversation flowed among the three upright caregivers and over the body of the bedridden Mrs. Smith. As the lights went on the instructor noticed a quiet, withdrawn woman sunken in a corner of the couch adjacent to the bed. The instructor left the group and walked over to her.

"Hello, my name is Ms. Ostralski and I am a nurse. I'm here with the students to care for Mrs. Smith. Are you a relative?"

"Yes, I'm her daughter, Mrs. Lanshen." She pulled herself up, became animated, and continued, "Do you know what is going to happen to my mother? She has been here 3 days, and I don't know anything."

"Do you live here in town?" the instructor inquired. At this point the students were getting squirmy, wondering when their instructor would finish this conversation and get back to the task for which they entered the room.

"Yes, we have lived here for years. However, Mother lived in a distant town until 3 weeks ago. We have just finished closing up her house and moving her here to live with us. Everything has been going well, until this. Now I just don't know what to do." She reached in her purse for a tissue and wiped the corners of her eyes as her voice became tremulous. "We finally thought we had things stabilized, and now this." Tears began to flow and the wide-eyed students observed their instructor to see what she would do next.

"Mrs. Lanshen, have you just come from work?" It was about 6:00 P.M. and she was well dressed.

"Yes, I have" she said, gaining composure. "I work full-time and I have Mom, and now I don't know what to do? Can I expect that she will get better? Will she have to go to a nursing home? Just think, only a few days ago we were talking about moving into a larger home so there would be more room for mother. Now this."

Mrs. Smith was 89 years old and like so many others in her age group, she had suffered a stroke. She was paralyzed on the left side of her body, incontinent of urine, and unable to feed herself without assistance. Her speech was intermittently incoherent and her activity curtailed. Within a brief period her daughter witnessed her vigorous, independent mother become feeble, dependent, and possibly on the verge of death. "Will she get better?" her daughter implored.

"Mrs. Lanshen, it is difficult to assess how your mother will progress. Generally, there is some improvement in the condition with time. She will require special care in the future. Have you thought about placing her in a nursing home?"

"Yes, I know one in our area, and my husband and I have discussed it."

"Good. I'm sure that once you have more facts from the medical team, you will be able to proceed by working with the Social Service Office here in this hospital. They will be able to assist you in making the necessary transport, admission, and financial arrangements. When that time draws closer, there will be someone to work with you specifically."

The instructor noticed how tired she appeared. "Mrs. Lanshen, I'll bet you haven't been home from work yet. Let us inquire about when the doctor will be here so you can talk to him."

"That would be great. I've been waiting for 2 days from after work until 8:00 P.M., and I haven't seen him yet. I could rest so much easier if I knew what to expect."

The instructor sent one of the students out only to discover that Mrs. Smith's doctor had gone home for the day. He had been in to see her before her daughter arrived. They relayed the information to her and told her they would inform the charge nurse, as well as place a note on her chart for the doctor to call her tomorrow. They procured her telephone number at home and at work and wrote a note to follow through with verbal and written communication.

Mrs. Lanshan stood up. "I feel so much better now. You are the first people to talk to me about Mom in two evenings. I feel she is in good hands so I can go now."

"Do go home and get some rest yourself now; we will take good care of your Mom." The instructor gave her a pat on the back as she discarded her tissue and gave us all a big smile.

"Thank you all," she said as she swiftly left the room closing the door behind her.

"Now," the instructor said to the students, "let us proceed with the neurological status exam."

Observations

Empathy, the capacity for participating in another's feelings or ideas, is an integral behavior of healers. Empathy should not be confused with sympathy, which means a relationship between people wherein whatever affects one similarly affects the other. During sympathy there is mutual or parallel susceptibility to the prevailing condition. Sympathy is not conducive to the healing process; empathy is.

Too often in the technological health-care delivery system empathy is abandoned or neglected in the cause of expediency. In the above situation the daughter and the mother are part and parcel of the same package. The mother may be in the bed, but the daughter requires as much, if not more, empathic attention to be healed.

The benefits of empathy are as follows:
- Increases the feeling of being connected to another
- Fosters self-esteem in those to whom you extend yourself
- Demonstrates to another that you genuinely accept them as they are
- Assists the other to increase self-awareness
- Allows the client to be less critical and increasingly caring toward themselves

ATTENTION TO DETAIL

When we attend to the details of care we make sure that all aspects are considered. As we become increasingly meticulous in caring for others, we will also note that organization and order improves in our own lives.

An Intravenous Therapy Nurse

"Take a deep breath and think of something pleasant. One, two, three, now," and with that Janice, with one quick, well-planned motion deeply thrust an 18-mm intravenous needle into the subclavian space just above her client's right collarbone. As Marsha lay silently on the bed Janice deftly threaded approximately 6 inches of sterile transparent filament into the vein she so skillfully entered. Within a period of seconds she connected the thread of tubing protruding from the chest to the prepared line coming from the liquid-filled plastic pouch on a stand above Marsha's bed. Just as quickly she procured a readied dressing complete with prophylactic antibiotic ointment and secured the entire apparatus snugly onto her client's chest. The next thing Marsha experienced was Janice whipping out her pen and writing the date, time, and her initials on a label. This way, she assured her client, anyone can tell at a glance when this procedure was started and the relative degree of freshness of the site, and when the topical dressing should be changed. This sounded good to Marsha, and it also felt as if Janice knew what she was doing.

Janice was an intravenous (I.V.) therapy nurse. For the past 11 years she has been one of eight nurses responsible for starting, maintaining, and properly terminating all the I.V.'s at Community Hospital. To get her job, Janice first became a R.N. with a firm knowledge of anatomy and physiology. She worked in a variety of staff nurse positions and became comfortable in dealing with several different personality types, fear levels, and pain thresholds. She became a confident, disciplined, and attentive caregiver. One day Janice read about I.V. therapy nurses at another hospital and decided to approach administration about the possibility of starting a program at Community Hospital. Much to her delight, and the patient's benefit, her proposal was accepted and Janice was given the position of organizing the I.V. Therapy Department. To do the best possible job Janice joined the Association of I.V. Therapy Nurses and after attending her first meeting she voraciously read everything she could on the topic and immediately began manipulative skill-building on plastic surrogate dummies. Within a few short weeks of her new appointment Janice was proficient with I.V.'s and ready to begin with patients using her new skills. Within 2 months she mastered several techniques and began an in-service program to teach four other nurses who had expressed interest in this new field. She wrote a curriculum, teaching objectives, and outcome criteria. She taught the classes, supervised the clinical practice, and determined who passed and who required more training. Janice was a stickler for detail. She knew skills were important, and so did the other nurses. One by one she built up the department until she had all three shifts covered all the time. It became known in the community—if you want expert nursing care, Community

Hospital offers it. The hospital infection rate decreased, and patient satisfaction increased.

Janice was low-keyed, not well known by her name, but a very important person who will be long remembered as a disciplined professional because of the skillful care rendered through attention to detail.

Observations

Attention to detail is a behavior common to healers. Without this attention procedures, techniques, and care rendered are inclined to be sloppy and fraught with flaws. Without attention to detail an important step in a procedure may be glossed over or inadvertently omitted altogether thereby rendering a technique or procedure that still might work but with increased hazards to the recipient. For example, if Janice were not attentive to, and expert at, each of the multistep details in her intravenous procedure, several things could happen. If her needle insertion technique was not mastered, then she could possibly cause more damage than cure as she probes for veins, contaminates the sterile field setting up a site for infection, and causes suffering to the unwary recipient of her services who is at her mercy. Because Janice believes that she is a nurse healer, she values the importance of her technical skill as a significant component of a healer's repertoire. She, and others like her, conscientiously practice and perfect skill building until it is tight and masterful. These healers recognize that attention to detail is an important part of their healing regime.

The benefits of details are as follows:
- Organizes our practice
- Assures an orderly completion of work
- Improves the odds of successful outcomes
- Provides a system for inclusion of all aspects of the endeavor

Healer Reflections

Have I identified my purpose in nursing?

How can I become more fully present as I interact with others?

Do I actively listen when others speak?

Are there ways I can employ empathy in my daily healing interventions?

Do I pay close attention to the details of care each time I perform a nursing-care skill?

Chapter 13

Expressions of Healing

If we are peaceful, if we are happy, we can smile and blossom like a flower, and everyone in our family, our entire society, will benefit from our peace.

Thich Nhat Hanh

Empowering Yourself

Note the many ways a healer can use their hands to soothe, comfort, and evoke another's own internal healing response.

Compare and contrast the various touch techniques.

Try to identify some of the counseling techniques you use from the many described in this chapter.

Compare and contrast the various counseling techniques used by nurse healers.

As you read the anecdotal story in expressions from the mind, think of circumstances in which you use your intellect in healing.

EXPRESSIONS THROUGH THE HANDS

Touch is probably one of our most highly used, yet least applauded, of the five recognized senses. It is the first sense to develop in the human embryo and the one most vital to survival.

We use touch in the literal sense in a myriad of ways ranging from the subtle fleeting brush stroke to heavy clapping percussion movements. Touch evokes the full range of emotions and often evokes our clients to release pent-up feelings.

As the largest sense organ of the body, the skin enables us to experience and learn about our environments. It is through the skin that the external world is perceived. The skin, particularly of the face, not only communicates to the brain the knowledge about the external world, but also conveys to others information about the state of a person's body, mind, and spirit.

Receiving Massage

"Lawrence, I don't think I can move. I'm so totally relaxed." Sally felt like she might melt directly into the table. "Must I get up?" Sally lay in pure luxury on the massage table. "I can't remember the last time I was this calm. What did you do to me?" Slowly and limply she raised herself and sat dangling her legs over the edge of the table as Lawrence went about some task just outside the curtain. Intellectually, she knew that the sensation of euphoria she was experiencing was the result of the physiological effects of the massage and she knew that the effects would last the rest of the day.

Observations

Deep muscle manipulation of several minutes' duration stimulates the release of endorphines, the body's own naturally occurring opiates. Documentation of this fact has given renewed credibility to nurses who practice bodywork therapies.

Hands-On Therapies

Hands on therapies have always been part of the healing process. Early in our history, shamans, wise women crones, laity and professionals alike, employed touch therapies. During the height of the Greek and Roman civilizations both hydrotherapy and massage were widely used. During the ensuing centuries health care providers continued to utilize massage until the advent of the scientific, technological revolution of the 1960s and 1970s. During these decades and those that followed, all health care therapies became subject to research scrutiny to ascertain true effectiveness and establish scientific credibility. Because there was no documented evidence of actual healing derived from touch therapies, their use dwindled to the extent that they became almost obsolete. For example, teaching students the practice of back massage was deleted from the curriculums of most nursing schools, the place where the skill had been taught and advocated since the mid-1800s when formal nurse training programs first began. During the mid-twentieth century the touch therapies were at their historic ebb. The West was still guided by its puritanical and technological heritage, and touch had yet to be documented as having any therapeutic validity.

During the 1980s, however, the touch therapies reemerged in force. Three events occurred to change the course history of this mode of healing. First, independent nurse practitioners developed their own specific and independent occupations based on hands-on healing. Second, scientific data documented measurable physical improvements correlated with body therapies; research studies showed physiological changes with touch. The third factor was the cross-culturalization of East and West. There was widespread Western interest in learning about the body therapies long used and accepted in the East. New therapies were developed as a result of a merger between the two cultural disciplines. As a result of these three events, public interest swelled as a renaissance in the body therapies began.

Today there is an enormous choice in varieties of body therapies ranging from physical tissue manipulation to energy field work to chakra center therapies. Table 13-1 details the major body therapies.

Table 13-1
Touch Therapy Modalities

- **Acupressure**: Based on the principle of acupuncture, practitioners of this ancient Chinese technique use finger pressure on specific points along body meridians to treat tension and stress, aches and pains, menstrual cramps or muscles strains, and arthritis. The system is also used for general preventative health care, warding off upper respiratory infections, improving muscle tone, and increasing energy levels.

- **Alexander Technique**: This technique was developed by an actor of the same name who created the method after concluding that bad posture was responsible for his own chronic voice loss. Practitioners teach simple, efficient movements designed to improve balance, posture, and coordination and to provide pain relief. Practitioners offer hands-on guidance and verbal instruction to retrain clients in the optimal use of their bodies.

- **Dance Movement Therapy**: In this modality expressive movement is used in a therapeutic way for both personal expression and psychological and emotional healing. Practitioners work with clients with physical disabilities, addiction problems, sexual abuse histories, eating disorders, and other concerns.

- **Deep Tissue Bodywork**: This is a general term for a range of therapies that work with the body's connective tissues and muscles to encourage them to function properly. Clients seek this therapy for whiplash, low back or neck pain, degenerative diseases, and preventive health maintenance.

- **Energy Field Work**: Practitioners in this field use their hands to sense weaknesses in the client's "energy field" that surrounds the body and seeks to restore its proper circulation and balance. Energy is channeled through the practitioner's hands and directed to strengthen the body's natural defenses to help the client's general state. This therapy may or may not include the physical laying on of hands. Visualization and discussion may also be used as part of the therapy.

- **Feldenkrais**: This modality combines movement training, touch, and discussion to assist clients to create freer, more efficient movement. Feldenkrais takes two forms. In individual hands-on sessions "Functional Integration," the practitioner's touch, is used to improve the subject's breathing and body alignment; and in a series of classes of slow, nonaerobic motions, "Awareness Through Movement," subjects "relearn" the proper ways their bodies should move. The method is frequently used to help reduce stress and tension, to alleviate chronic pain, and to help athletes and others improve their balance and coordination.

- **Hellerwork**: Developed by a former aerospace engineer, this technique combines deep-tissue muscle therapy and movement reeducation with dialogue about the emotional issues that may underlie physical posture. For example, feelings of insecurity may manifest themselves in stooped shoulders. Participants go through eleven 60- to 90-minute sessions. The first session, "Inspiration," addresses the rib cage area and focuses on breathing. Stressing the body-mind connection, Hellerwork is used to treat chronic pain or to help well clients learn to live more comfortably in their bodies.

- **Infant Massage**: Taught to new parents by trained instructors, infant massage practices are designed to enhance the bonding between parent and child. As preventive therapy, infant massage can help strengthen and regulate a baby's respiratory, circulatory, and gastrointestinal functions, often relieving gas and colic while relaxing both parent and child.

- **Jin Shin Jyutsu**: This oriental system is intended to harmonize the flow of energy through the body. The underlying belief is that tension, fatigue, or illness can trap energy in the body's twenty-six "safety energy locks." Practitioners use their hands to restore balance and reduce stress. Jin Shin Jyutsu is not a form of massage since it does not involve physical manipulation of the muscles.

- **Kinesiology**: This is a diagnostic system based on the premise that individual muscle functions can be used to provide information about a client's overall health. Practitioners test the strength and mobility of certain muscles, analyze a client's posture and gait, and inquire about life-style factors that may be contributing to an illness. The theory is that if muscles are strong, then circulation and other vital functions are also strong. Nutrition, muscle and joint manipulation, diet, and exercise may then be used as part of a treatment plan.

- **Kofutu Touch Healing**: This system was developed in the early 1970s when a series of symbols for use in touch came to the originator during meditation. It is called "Kofute" for the symbols and "touch" healing because the auras of the healer and recipient must touch. This therapy uses higher consciousness energy symbols for the purpose of self-development and spiritual healing.

- **Massage Therapy**: This is a general term for a range of therapeutic approaches with roots in both Eastern and Western cultures. It involves the practice of kneading or otherwise manipulating a person's muscles and other soft tissue with the intent of improving the client's well-being and health.

- **Neuromuscular Therapy**: This therapy emphasizes the role of the brain, spine, and nerves in muscular pain. One goal of the therapy is to relieve tender congested spots in muscle tissue and compressed nerves that may radiate pain to other areas of the body.

- **Ohashiatsu**: This is a system of physical techniques, exercise, and meditation used to relieve tension and fatigue and induce a state of harmony and peace. The practitioner first assesses a person's state of "hara" (the area below the navel). Then, using continuous and flowing movements, the practitioner presses and stresses the body's energy channels, working in unison with the person's breathing.

- **Orthobionomy**: This technique involves the use of noninvasive, gentle touch along with dialogue and instruction in common movements such as walking, sitting, standing, and reaching. Practitioners may also work with the energy field surrounding the person. The goal of this therapy is to enhance the client's well-being and empowerment, rather than physical healing.

- **Polarity**: This system holds that energy fields and currents exist throughout nature and that the flow and balance of this energy in the human body is the underlying foundation of health. In a polarity session, the practitioner may use bodywork and guidance in diet, exercise, and life-style to help balance this energy, release blocked energy, and support healing.

- **Reflexology**: Specific points on the hands and feet correspond with organs and tissues throughout the body. With fingers and thumbs, the practitioner applies pressure to these points to treat a wide range of stress-related illnesses and ailments.

- **Reiki**: Practitioners of this ancient Tibetan healing system use light hand placements to channel healing energies to the recipient. Practitioners vary widely in technique and philosophy, yet all use the system to treat emotional and mental distress, chronic and acute problems, and to assist the recipient in achieving spiritual focus and clarity.

- **Rolfing**: This technique uses deep manipulation of the fascia (connective tissue) to restore the body's natural alignment, which may become rigid through injury, emotional trauma, and inefficient movement habits. The process involves ten sessions, each focusing on a different part of the body.

- **Rosen Method**: This technique combines gentle touch with verbal communication to evoke emotion with the goal of achieving relaxation and self-awareness.

- **Shiatsu**: A form of Japanese acupressure, this practice has been used for more than 1000 years to treat pain and illness and for general health maintenance. Practitioners use a series of techniques to apply rhythmic finger pressure at specific points on the body to stimulate "chi," which is considered vital energy.

- **Structural Integration**: This is a systematic approach to relieving patterns of stress and impaired functioning. This therapy seeks to correct misalignments in the body created by gravity and physical and psychological trauma. In a series of ten sessions the practitioner uses hands, arms, and elbows to apply pressure to the connective tissue while the client participates through directed breathing techniques.

- **Therapeutic Touch**: This practice is based on the premise that the body is an open system of energies that are in constant flux and that illness is caused by a deficit or an imbalance of these energies. The TT practitioner "assesses" where the person's field is weak or congested, and then uses the hands to direct energy into the field to balance it.

- **Touch for Health**: This is a system of balancing the body's energy by applying gentle pressure to contracted muscles and other points along the body. Regular balancing is used to improve overall health and strengthen resistance to common ailments and physical complaints.

- **Trager**: This technique uses rocking and shaking to loosen the joints and ease movement. During the session the practitioner cradles and moves the client's still limbs to retrain the body's old patterns of movement and prevent problems from recurring.

- **Trigger Point/Myotherapy**: Practitioners of this modality apply pressure to specific points on the body to relieve tension. Trigger points are tender, congested spots on muscle tissue that may radiate pain to other areas. Though the technique is similar to shiatsu or acupressure, this therapy uses Western anatomy and physiology as its basis.

- **Yoga**: Yoga is a general term for a range of body-mind exercises used to access consciousness and encourage physical and mental well-being. Some forms concentrate on achieving perfection in posture and alignment of the physical body; others aim at mental control to access higher consciousness. Still other forms focus on the varying relationships of body, mind, spirit, and energy.

When a nurse chooses to utilize this healing modality, he or she must first ask, do I like to touch or be touched? Do I believe that healing power can flow through me, spirit to mind, mind to hands, and from my hands to another's being? Do I want to help other people in this way? If the answers are affirmative, then choose to connect to others with the healing power of touch.

EXPRESSIONS FROM THE HEAD

It was a warm spring afternoon when June was busily working at home and the ring of the telephone interrupted her. It was her neighbor, who because she was crying so hard, could barely talk. She did manage to convey she was in need, and could June please drop what she was doing and come right over. Since she was not the kind of person to bother others without cause, June stopped her work and rushed over. Her neighbor's tear-stained face indicated whatever was troubling her was immense. Without much articulation her trembling hand thrust a torn out newspaper page into June's hand and she simply said, "Read this."

"Heart Doctor Discusses Heart Disease;" the newspapers date was today. Realizing that no one had died and that she was in no immediate danger, June moved to sit down. She chose the living room couch and pulled Barb along to sit close beside her. June turned and propped herself up against the side cushion turning toward the center of the couch so that she could both read the article and face Barb simultaneously. June sensed Barb would be studying her for a reaction. Barb positioned herself facing June and watched her face for her response as she carefully read the article. It turned out to be about the diagnosis, treatment, and prognosis of myocarditis, a viral inflammation of the heart muscle.

Barb, age 47, had been diagnosed 10 months earlier with myocarditis. The key sentence in the paper that was apparently responsible for her consternation was the sentence, "the only possible outcome of myocarditis is death or heart transplant."

Barb's eyes searched June as she finished reading. It was clear to June that Barb believed that the news article was written directly to and about her and that she was going to die. Here at last sat her healer friend, what she would say would determine her final reaction? She waited for June to confirm the verdict. June knew that the words she chose, the movements she made, and the expression on her face all mattered. Barb was receptive to every nuance. She trusted June and had sought her out for advice before; she would match June's response. June was the one after all who said in the first place that she must have a medical examination to determine the cause of her chest pain. Now 10 months later, the seriousness of her ailment had abruptly become apparent to both of them.

June began her initial response slowly, without display of emotion. "Now first of all Barb, I want you to realize that newspapers sensationalize. You need to know that there are other options that the reporter simply did not include. There is always the possibility of recovery. Obviously, this reporter wanted to be dramatic and omitted that possibility. Heart muscle can heal, you know people who have recovered from heart attacks." By this time Barb had stopped sobbing, took some deep breaths, and continued to stare expectantly at June. She continued, "the second thing is, has your cardiologist told you that this was a fatal condition?"

"Not exactly," Barb replied. "He did say, however, that if I did not lose this weight, it could kill me."

June decided she must address the weight issue, but that first she would discuss the primary emotion that the article stimulated. June felt the need to confront Barb about her own mortality. "Barb, the other thing that seems to have you upset is the possibility of dying." She sat silently waiting for me to continue. "It is important to remember that we all die sometime. The impact of this article offers you an opportunity to stop and reflect just how you are living each and every day. You know we have talked about this before—remember when Mrs. Reinowski down the street died last year in an automobile accident. She was only 40. None of us know when or where our life will end, and because of that, we need to become increasingly conscious of how we live each and every day. Are you living each day as if it might be your last?" As June expected, the tears poured forth again and her real fears surfaced. At this point June moved forward and held Barb as she cried. In addition to the empathy June felt, she knew that new research has found that tears contain hormones. It is theorized that these hormones rid the body of harmful emotions during a tearing episode. Consequently, June did not say anything, but rather rocked her and let her cry. Soon enough she finished, and leaned back looking exhausted. June decided to let the death issue alone. It had been brought to the surface, and now she required time to process it. However, determined not to let go of the power of the moment, June decided to move ahead to plan some concrete strategies.

"Now," June said, "let's talk about the weight problem." Without hesitating she launched right in, "Tell me your weight." Anyone with a weight problem knows that is not a question that a friend should ever ask. That is private and confidential information. Barb hesitated, looking coy. "Tell me how much you weigh," June said again. Barb stammered around, she began telling June how much she had weighed when pregnant and how much more than that she weighed now. "Tell me how many pounds you are now." At this point June was persistent and demanding. She sincerely believed that Barb must state the facts and take a hard, cold look at them before she could proceed with helping Barb evoke her own internal healing resources.

Finally Barb looked at June and said, "212 pounds." Without flinching and with no emotional display June replied, "And what is your ideal body weight?"

Barb began to relax again, "With my large frame and height, my ideal weight is around 150 pounds." Now armed with the facts and more importantly her enunciation of them, June felt they could proceed to deal with the weight issue from an intellectual, as well as an emotional, basis.

"Barb, you are fat. Do you realize you are fat?" The word fat stung as the issue began to emotionally sink in. "Barb, tell me you are fat."

She retorted, "I can't say it."

"Yes," June replied, "you can. Barb, tell me what you are."

Again the tears, yet through them came her voice, sobbing yet sure, "I am fat." With increasing force she said, "I am fat," three more times. We both were quiet after that, and I hugged her until the crying subsided. It was at this point that the breakthrough was made. Barb had acknowledged her fear of dying, her weight problem, and the fact she needed more information about her medical condition.

The behaviors of detached compassion (listening without becoming emotionally involved), perseverance (achieving the goal of her acknowledgment of the problem despite the difficulty), and the attitudes of driving toward a sense of purpose and caring for her were present throughout this interaction.

"Okay, Barb, let's talk about where you go from here." At this point they moved immediately to constructive planning for a weight-loss program. June illustrated the size of the heart muscle by showing her a clinched fist and told her to imagine trying to lift an extra 60 pounds. "Just think of the poor little heart trying to pump so much harder to supply nourishment to all that extra weight." After she had identified with this analogy by making her own fist and pointing to the imaginary pile of pounds beside her, she was ready to move ahead. After some dialogue it was her decision to begin Weight Watchers again that very evening.

June had previously talked to her about affirmations regarding another issue, so it was not new territory when she said, "Let's write some specific affirmations." June told her to go get a pencil and paper and return. She came sprinting back, quickly nestled in again on the couch and began writing as together they worked out six affirmation statements about the positive effect of her weight loss and her increasingly effective cardiac muscle. After June left, she would type the affirmations on three separate cards: one for her bathroom mirror, the second for the refrigerator door, and the third to carry with her in her purse wherever she went. By this time she was genuinely excited about doing the statements.

Barb was scheduled to receive an allergy injection at her general practitioner's office in 2 days. Because both of them felt she needed some reassurance from her physician, June suggested she call the clinic in advance and ask for time to speak with the doctor at the time of her injection. June hoped the physician would proceed in a similar manner to her response.

Observations

This example illustrates how in one unexpected encounter a healer can evoke and unlock powerful inner healer resources in another. In this case it took the combination of compassion, empathy, listening, knowledge, discipline, goal setting, and love. These are some of the attributes of a healer. They are not elusive, unobtainable traits but rather behaviors available to anyone who desires to become a healer.

Today nurses have a wealth of counseling modalities to choose from. Table 13-2 details some of them.

Table 13-2
Nurse Counseling Modalities

- **Bioenergetics**: The theory behind this modality is that repressed emotions and desires affect the body, mind, and spirit by creating chronic muscular tension and diminished vitality and energy. Through verbal therapy the nurse guides the client to use physical exercise, breathing techniques, psychotherapy, and other forms of emotional-release work to loosen the clients "character armor" and restore natural well-being.

- **Biofeedback**: This is a counseling technique used especially for stress-related conditions such as insomnia, migraine headaches, and hypertension. In biofeedback sensitive, monitoring machines measure skin temperature, heart rate, and muscle tension to give "biological feedback" to the client. By consciously visualizing, relaxing, or imagining while observing light, sound, or verbal guidance, the client learns to make subtle adjustments to move toward a more balanced internal state.

- **Body-Centered Psychotherapy**: Practitioners of this therapy believe that emotional issues and past trauma are experienced through the body. For example, unresolved conflict on the job may be transferred to shoulder and neck muscle tightening with resultant migraine headaches. Body-centered psychotherapy uses physical sensations as a reference point in exploring these issues.

- **Focusing**: This therapy is based on the premise that information about one's life issues can be accessed through the physical body. The nurse therapist assists the client to focus on these "felt senses" for greater understanding and to reach resolution. The issues addressed include such areas as decision making, recovery from abuse, enhancing creativity, and improving the body-mind functioning.

- **Hypnotherapy**: This refers to a range of techniques that allow practitioners to bypass the conscious mind and access the subconscious where suppressed memories, repressed emotions, and forgotten events remain recorded. Some psychiatric nurse healers use this technique for smoking cessation, weight loss programs, phobias, and general stress management.

- **Rebirthing**: The therapist guides clients through a series of breathing exercises to help them reexperience past memories. The focus centers around the actual birth experience with the intent to assist the client to let go of emotional tensions long stored in the body and to rebirth to new health and vitality.

- **Stress management**: This therapy encompasses a broad range of modalities designed to address the mental, emotional, and physical results of accumulated stress. Approaches include counseling, bodywork, life-style behavior restructuring, meditation, prayer, energy work, and education.

EXPRESSIONS OF THE SPIRIT

"Close your eyes now, and repeat these words with me. I am relaxed, . . . I am still . . . , I am receptive and willing to have the flow of healing energy enter my being. Now while in silent concentration allow your mind and spirit to concentrate on the energy that surrounds and lights your being."

John stood before the three of us, hands outstretched, eyes closed, and face uplifted. "Mighty Lord, fill me with the spirit, that I may be a channel for healing. Open my heart and begin the flow of healing energy to soothe the ills of these suffering ones."

Briefly opening his eyes, John moved to stand before Tim. "You have declared the pain of loss. Someone close to you has made the transition from earth. Since that time you have suffered pain in your chest." He gazed into Tim's upturned face. Closing his eyes again he continued, pray with me now and allow the Holy Spirit to fill you." Tim saw his open palms a few inches from his face as he gently shut his eyes and moved into the space of his rhythmic expression.

"Great source of life and healing, focus on this man in his time of need. Send your spirit to engage his own. Allow him to feel the warmth and comfort of divinity. I pray that you guide and assist him during his time of sorrow. Fill his heart with gladness and thanksgiving and help him heal." His voice flowed on as Tim knelt in wonder before this heretofore unknown man who was so completely present in his life at this moment. He became absorbed in this self-selected activity. The longer he spoke, the more centered and present Tim became.

"I feel warmth and tingling in my chest. My hands are so warm, my body so relaxed. Yes, I do want to be healed. Come to me and enter my being. Help me to be better." Tim began to utter these words spontaneously and without prompting. This was most unlike him. Yet something was happening, here and now, his physical being felt penetrated by spirit. Without further articulation, Tim knew he would be better. Here in a stranger's living room something most extraordinary happened to him, he felt genuinely engaged by spirit.

Following the session Tim returned to a state of analytical inquiry. Was it the placebo effect? It was his curiosity that drew him to explore this phenomenon. He came with two friends for a first-hand experience with a nurse who had merged his nursing knowledge with his intuitive spiritual insights and had emerged as a reputed psychic, known for his healing ability. Did his healing work? At this point in time instruments for measuring the effectiveness of spiritual healing are still in the developmental stage. When attempting to validate healings we can only ask, does the recipient feel better, do they get well? In this case Tim certainly experienced relief. All three of them left John's house a bit mystified, but feeling stronger than when they arrived. They were optimistic that soon Tim would be symptom free.

Spiritual Healing

What is spiritual healing? Does it really work? If so, who and what kind of people subscribe to it? Spiritual healers believe it is not they who do the healing. Rather they serve as channels for the healing power that comes from God or a source beyond themselves. The goal of a spiritual healer is to become a clearer channel, which means overcoming obstructions such as greed, resentment, pride, and egotism. One continually works to overcome these traits.

The mind is amenable to suggestion. Some believe that in a deep sleep or trance state the subconscious mind has the power to interpret the objective mind of others. It can acquire or intuit from the subconscious mind of other individuals operating on the same frequency. The subconscious mind forgets nothing. The conscious mind receives the impression from without and transfers all thought to the subconscious where it remains even though the conscious mind may be destroyed. The subconscious mind is in direct communication with all other subconscious minds and is able to gather all the knowledge possessed by millions of other subconscious minds. Some refer to this phenomenon as tapping into the Akashic Records. The term Akashic is a mystical and allegorical one. It refers to the indelible record of all events, occurrences, and knowledge, which is an integral part of the cosmic consciousness. All things that have come to pass or that will happen are established in the Akashic Records. Some believe that by focused intent they can attune with cosmic consciousness and be imbued with its omniscience. The word Akashic is derived from the Sanskrit word, Akasa, which means an indeterminate essence such as space ether.

During the healing process you open yourself up to God or a higher power. The key to accomplishing this is found through quieting, centering, and focused attention. During this state of being you allow the healing power to flow through you to the ill or troubled person. Some spiritual healers work with the assistance of "helpers." These helpers include angels, inner guides, power animals, the client's higher self, or other spiritual forces. The practitioner may think of himself or herself as a priest/priestess, shaman, wise woman, or soul retriever. The spiritual healer does not claim to be responsible for the healing, but believes that he or she is a conduit for healing energy from the spiritual realm.

Edgar Cayce

Edgar Cayce, a renown spiritual healer during the 1930s and 1940s, commented on some of the key questions regarding spiritual healing. Today there are several medical clinics that still follow his guidelines and incorporate several of his healing techniques. The Association for Research and Enlightenment (ARE) is a foundation that supports research and education in this area.

Cayce responded as follows to these questions: How do you open yourself to God? Answer, "In meditation and with the aid of breathing exercises you attune the inner self to a consciousness of the oneness of the individual life with Universal Consciousness. Through this attunement, the body's vibrations will begin to rise. The body then becomes like a magnet as spirit answers to spirit."

What factors help or hinder the flow? Answer, "In order to raise the body's vibrations high enough so that they flow out of self to the person for whom healing is intended, there must be a unity of purpose in the group. Each member should look into himself and overcome attitudes such as cynicism, selfishness, envy, and resentment and develop virtues such as love and patience and the desire to be of service to others. In other words, one must heal oneself in order to heal others, but conversely, one heals himself by healing others. It helps to feel oneself surrounded by divine love while healing."

How is the healing power conveyed to the ill person? Answer, "The vibrations raised in the body are emanations of the life force from within and are material expressions of a spiritual influence. The spiritualized emanations are sent out through the pituitary gland as thought waves, by suggestive force, or by visualizing the healing activity on the ill person."

What attitude is best for the person receiving the healing? Answer, "The ill person should seek help and have a sincere desire to be healed. It is best if he has faith that he will be healed and if he cooperates wholeheartedly with the healer by coordinating his meditation and prayers with theirs so that his consciousness will be raised at the same time."

Other Spiritual Healers

Most spiritual healers believe you have to purify yourself and reach a state of attunement by giving an affirmation or saying a prayer. Words such as, "let only good pass through me to the client" are important to think or articulate before proceeding to the healing act. You put yourself aside; your mood is passive and receptive. You think of power coming down through the top of your head and down through your hands.

In magnetic healing in which you take deep breaths, forcing the healing energy out, the energy seems to come from the healer and leaves him spent, but when you think of yourself as a channel, the healing gives you a sense of strength.

Catherine, a nurse, relates how she became a healer. "I sensed I had the ability to heal when I was a child. People said they felt soothed and relaxed when I was present. I developed this by continuous use and by concentrating on opening myself to the psychic flow of the healing power. It continues to grow within me. Now I do the laying on of hands. I place my hands 3 or 4 inches away from the body. I invoke the God force through prayer, asking if it is the God force's will for the person to be healed and, if so, for the betterment of the person. You merely ask to be a channel of God's healing".

Spiritual and mental preparation for healing involves prayer and concentration to evoke the energy flow from mind to hands. Too often people are solely interested in the body, not the soul, too obsessed with how and not enough concerned with the why of it. Many people seldom question why they are ill. Yet, most illness has an origin in the spirit or mind, as well as the physical body. Consequently, nurse healers will want to consider the spirit and mind as they give attention to the physical body.

It is good to state affirmations. These are spiritual truths that, when articulated, uplift the soul. If beliefs are negative, they may materialize in discomfort and disease. However, if they are positive, good, and wholehearted, then they probably will materialize as comfort and healing.

To stimulate a response in a sick person, the healer's thoughts or prayers should be clear and purposeful. On the other hand, to respond to another person's healing or prayers, the sick person should be convinced of the healer's goodwill.

Some believe that healing occurs when there is self-attunement to the Source of all healing power and energy. Connection with the spirit seems to be a matter of raising one's vibrations to a state that enables the reception the spiritual energy. With focus or concentration, as well as intent, this is a practice that is available to us all. By our thoughts we have the ability to become cocreators with the universal spirit, and it is with the spirit that we most effectively function as nurse healers.

Healer Reflections

Do I like to use my hands in healing?

Do I believe that healing power can flow through me, mind to mind, mind to hands, and from my hands to heal others?

When I touch with intention, what is my inner experience?

Is it possible that each of us is part of a Universal Source and that I have some of this source whenever I perform a creative act?

Who do I know who can be my mentor to help me increase my expressive healing skills?

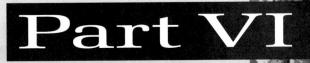

Part VI

Complementary Nurse Healer Modalities

The first step in the evolution of a nurse healer is to understand the importance of developing empowering attitudes and behaviors. The next level involves becoming familiar with some of the independent nursing therapies available to nurse healers. There are numerous therapeutic modalities available to the nurse healer. The few highlighted in this section include the following:

- Breathing and relaxation
- Visualization and imagery
- Meditation and prayer
- Music

Each of the therapies can be used alone or coupled with one another. Once the skills are mastered, you may want to use them in various combinations for greater effect.

The following chapters will guide you to increasing awareness of selected healing modalities that nurse healers can utilize both for themselves and with clients in daily nursing practice.

Chapter 14

Breathing and Relaxation

Empowering Yourself

Become aware of how breathing and relaxation allows you to feel a sense of timelessness.

Know that when you feel timelessness, your concerns about the issues at hand melt into a sense of greater perspective.

Note that relaxation requires time to learn. Even though the concept seems simple, practice sessions are necessary to master the skill.

Consider that when you learn these skills, you will increase your ability to release stresses and tensions.

REACTION TO LIFE'S STRESSORS

Before you read this chapter, pause, take a deep breath, and then go look in the mirror. What do you see? Are your facial muscles relaxed and smooth, or do you have furrows and creases that demarcate worry, stress, and hurry?

Often this simple mirror exercise can yield valuable feedback about the effects of our internal state of body-mind balance or imbalance. There is no question that nursing is a stressful occupation that, when added to the usual stresses of daily living in the fast-paced, contemporary world, causes most nurses to carry heavy loads of internalized tensions. Among other things, accumulated stress can block the flow of valuable energy and put the nurse in the position of minimizing interpersonal relationships with clients and colleagues.

As you read this chapter you will discover how to use breathing and relaxation to release the tension first in yourself and then to transfer that learning to the patient-care arena. When you master the art of relaxed, peak performance, then you will be in an excellent position to (1) assist your clients to breathe and relax as they undergo health-care challenges, and (2) to teach them skills that can assist them in the prevention of stress-related illnesses.

EVOKING THE RELAXATION RESPONSE

Many scholars have named and described ways to relax. Some techniques and the theorists who developed them include the following:
- Breathe work—Stansolof Groff
- Autogenics—J.H. Schultz
- Autosuggestion—Emil Coue
- Progressive relaxation—Edmund Jacobson
- Biofeedback—Elmer Green
- Biogenics—C. Norman Shealy
- Relaxation response—Herbert Benson

Breathing

Most people take breathing for granted. Others, however, such as singers, actors, public speakers, and some nurse healers know that there is more to breathing than the involuntary, lifelong, repetitive act of diaphragmatic inspiration and expiration.

By employing conscious breathing skills you can improve circulation, enhance thinking, and even affect muscle tone. Some forms of yoga focus entirely on the development of the interplay between breathing, consciousness, and movement. Nurse healers will want to explore some breathing techniques both for themselves and their clients.

Breathing Exercise

Follow the steps in this exercise to experience the realm of conscious breathing.

1. Sit comfortably in a chair with both feet flat on the ground. Allow your arms to rest comfortably at your side or on the table. When you guide someone else, ask them to close their eyes and follow the direction of your voice.

2. Take a deep inspiration, and then exhale. Repeat to yourself as you read or listen:
   I breathe in. I breathe out.
   I breathe in. I breathe out.
   I breathe in. I breathe out.

3. Begin to consciously feel the inhaled breath swirling around in your body gathering up the toxins to eliminate during the slow, deliberate exhalation. Repeat to yourself as you proceed:
   I breathe in clean, healing air.
   I exhale toxins and tensions.
   I breathe in clean, healing air.
   I exhale toxins and tensions.
   I breathe in clean, healing air.
   I exhale toxins and tensions.

4. As you continue to grow in awareness of your breathing, feel the nostrils flare with your inhalation and relax during exhalation. Repeat to yourself as you proceed:
   I breathe in. I breathe out.
   I breathe in. I breathe out.
   I breathe in. I breathe out.

5. As you breathe, feel the clean, fresh air begin to circulate throughout your body picking up old, stale air for removal during exhalation. Again focus on the flaring of your nostrils as you inhale. At this point allow your lips to gently part as you exhale the stale air through your mouth.

Repeat to yourself as you proceed:
    Fresh, clean air energizes me.
    My tension is released as I exhale.
    Fresh, clean air energizes me.
    My tension is released as I exhale.

6. Realize at this point that your breathing is effortless and calming. Think of a single word that epitomizes wholeness and unity to you. The word might be "om," "one," "peace," "unity," or some other significant word to you. For the next several breaths think of this word as you exhale. Now repeat to yourself as you do it:
    I breathe in. I breathe out.
    Think of your word as you exhale.
    I breathe in. I breathe out.
    Think of your word as you exhale.
    I breathe in. I breathe out.
    Think of your word as you exhale.

7. As you conclude this series of repetitions, allow the word to float away as if drifting on a puffy, white cloud in an azure blue sky. Repeat these phrases:
    I breathe effortlessly and easily.
    I am relaxed.
    I breathe effortlessly and easily.
    I am relaxed.
    I breathe effortlessly and easily.
    I am relaxed.

8. Slowly and gently bring your awareness back to the place and setting where you are, and if your eyes were closed, open them.

Optimally this exercise should last 10 or more minutes. With increased time the participant should be directed to image fresh, invigorating air cleansing of all organ systems and muscle groups in the body.

Implementing the Exercise

After you experience the beneficial results, you will want to use breathing techniques with your clients. The clinical arena is full of opportunities to utilize this skill. Obstetric nurses already know the value of focused breathing for women during active labor. It has been the focus of Lamaze childbirth techniques for decades. Most clients in compromised, clinical situations will benefit from the nurse healer who can guide them through focused breathing techniques.

Preoperative and postoperative patients, children awaiting immunizations, and those undergoing outpatient procedures are just some of the acute-care clients who can benefit from simple breathing exercises. The use of breathing techniques are a natural when working with clients in counseling, touch therapy, or preventive care. When mastered, an individual can use breathing techniques to alter both physiology and emotions.

Relaxation

Breathing and relaxation go hand in hand. It is difficult to fully relax without slowing and deepening our breathing. For example, when we go to sleep the body naturally relaxes and breathing deepens and slows. Genuine relaxation involves slowing and balancing the body, mind, and spirit. The kind of relaxation that refreshes and invigorates comes from moving away from the busy, working world and entering a space of quietness and inner reflection. While the passive activity of watching television may seem relaxing, program content will affect whether we relax. In most cases regular programing stimulates us with dilemmas, conflict, or violence. Often program content will carry over into problem solving that goes on unconsciously at night during the dream period. For this reason one should carefully select television programs, especially when trying to relax.

Relaxation reduces the body's oxygen consumption, heart rate, respiratory rate, metabolism, blood pressure, and increases alpha brain waves. All these physiologic responses promote a sense of well-being that includes mental calming and emotional balance.

Types of Relaxation

Two widely recognized methods of relaxation are as follows:

1. Progressive muscle relaxation developed by Jacobson in 1938. This technique involves the contraction and relaxation of specific muscle groups.

2. Relaxation response developed by Benson in 1975. To evoke the relaxation response one needs the following four elements:
   - A quiet environment
   - An object on which to dwell
   - A passive attitude
   - A comfortable position

Progressive Relaxation Exercise

Settle comfortably in a chair with your feet flat on the ground. Repeat to yourself or read aloud the following and use as a guide when assisting clients through this exercise:

I tighten my right fist. I feel my fist tighter and tighter and study the tension as I do so.

I allow the muscles in my right fist to loosen, and as they relax, I observe the contrast in my feelings.

Once again I tighten my right fist. As I hold it, I notice the tension again.

I let go of the tension in my right fist, I straighten my fingers and notice the difference I feel.

I repeat the exercise with my left fist.

I tighten my left fist as the rest of my body relaxes.

I allow the muscles in my left fist to loosen, and as they relax, I observe the contrast in the sensations.

I repeat the tightening and relaxing exercise in my left fist.

Again, I enjoy the contrast.

Now I tighten the muscles in both fists and feel the tension.

Now I fully relax and enjoy the sensation.

I tighten the muscles in both fists, and both arms. I observe the feeling in my arms.

I allow the muscles in both arms and wrists to relax and feel the sensation of relaxation rippling through me.

Each muscle group in the body is progressively tightened and relaxed as the participant's mental focus remains on the process. As the experience continues, the participant should couple deep breathing along with the progressive relaxation. The entire exercise should last a minimum of 10 minutes and cover all the major muscles groups of the body. At the conclusion of the exercise the client is invariably physically relaxed, and the emotions are balanced. In settings where the client can sleep following this exercise, sleep is often deep and restful.

Implementing the Exercise

Progressive relaxation can be used by nurse healers in any clinical setting. Imagine yourself in an acute care setting with an anxious patient. If you can create a period of 10 minutes to spend with your client, think of the benefit you can offer to someone receptive to this modality. In gerontology or pediatric settings try this technique instead of offering sleeping medications. You will be surprised how effectively it works.

The Relaxation Response

Active nurse healers are prime candidates for following the steps to evoke the relaxation response on themselves. Since you are busy and focused on others during much of the working period, you will naturally accumulate tensions. Since you are aware of the results of accumulated stress, you will want to rid yourself of collected tensions from time to time. The four-point program of Benson's technique can be done anywhere. Optimally, of course, it would be nice to go somewhere outside the workplace, but since this is not usually possible, try to follow the four-step process wherever you are.

1. Find a quiet environment. Easier said than done, you say. If you are in a large, acute-care setting, have you tried the institution's chapel? Usually the chapel is empty and easily accessible to nurses. It is quiet, and the following three steps readily flow from this setting.

   If you work in an intensive care area, the most private place you can find may be the rest room. Go there or to the break room to get away from a chaotic environment and to sit and be quiet for a few minutes.

2. Use an object on which to dwell. You may want to carry a small talisman with you in your pocket, or if not, focus on an object such as a pastoral painting on an opposite wall.

3. Assume a passive attitude. Do this as you focus on your breathing and muscle relaxation. Allow your worries and stressors of the preceding moments to pass through and out of your mind. Release attachment to the troublesome or irritating thoughts that bother you. Remember that they are but passing instances in a spectrum, dimension, or domain that encompasses the whole of life. Use this time to put your immediate concerns in perspective.

4. Sit in a comfortable position. Make sure that your back is straight or supported and that your limbs are in a loose, relaxed position as you focus on your breathing, relaxation, and calm thinking.

After you practice the relaxation response in private, eventually you will be able to evoke it even in the midst of crisis. Relaxation is primarily a mental exercise and once mastered, can be evoked in any setting. It is an excellent tool to carry in your mental purse wherever you go.

Healer Reflections

As I practice the skill of deep breathing, am I able to focus on the act of inspiration and expiration and exclude external, troubling thoughts?

Can I actually feel the rush of cleansing air fill my physical body as I practice the breathing exercise?

Am I aware of the release of physical, mental, and emotional tensions when I concentrate on tightening and releasing muscle groups during the progressive relaxation exercise?

Where can I go in my work setting to continue to practice the evocation of the relaxation response?

Chapter 15

Visualization and Imagery

Empowering Yourself

Know that imagery allows you to create mental pictures that your holistic being can manifest on the physical plane.

Recognize that visualization has to do with achieving positive end results.

Consider that imagery is a skill that has been practiced for centuries by healers.

Think of visualization and imagery as a key to unlock the door to an effective healing skill.

Anticipate that imagery is a good way to learn more about the potential of your creative healing ability.

AWAKENING THE CREATIVE MIND

The technique of visualization or imagery assists you to awaken or refine your ability to create powerful, mental pictures. This internal process involves opening the mind to mental ideas of positive, creative images that can foster self-healing, as well as present and future successes. Images can be evoked from our memories, fantasies, hopes, and dreams. An individual experienced in imagery can employ all the senses to actually hear, see, feel, touch, or even taste the created image. When doing this, a holistic connection of body, mind, and spirit is made.

The Goal of Visualization and Imagery

The goal of this healing modality is to create a mental picture or series of pictures that depict how you or your client want things to be. For example, you as a nurse healer may want to evoke images of being healthy, physically fit, mentally alert, emotionally balanced, and spiritually attuned. As you move through the realm of linear time, the process of achieving your goals will be hastened when you use the process of imagery to create and hold fast to the desired end result.

Learning the Process

The ability to effectively image and visualize can be learned either individually through self-direction or by the guided-imagery process. This modality, like previous ones, should be mastered first by the nurse and then used with clients.

IMAGERY EXERCISES

The ability to practice imagery skills flows naturally from the previously discussed skills of breathing and relaxation. You may have heard the old expression, "be careful what you ask for, because you may get it." Our images are so powerful that they do indeed create our future. Many of us are unconscious of the fact that we image all the time, and the pictures we project and the words we say combine to actually create our reality. It is when we become conscious of the process that we can develop the ability to mold and shape our images and thoughts to create a healthy, positive destiny. Once you experience the power of this modality, you will likely commit to utilizing this skill in your own life, as well as in your healing practice.

There are numerous techniques to hasten the development of your ability to image. They include exercises in seeing colors, images, yourself, your inner guide, and/or your goals and desires. Sample a few exercises here and now.

Smelling the Roses

- Position yourself comfortably, loosen tight clothing, and allow your arms to be gently supported.
- Imagine yourself in a beautiful, well-kept garden. See yourself sitting in the middle of the garden in a comfortable patio chair with your feet supported on an ottoman.
- Look around you and see the manicured box hedges and well-designed arrangement of ornamental, flowering, dogwood trees and hanging, fucia-colored bougainvillea.
- Feel the warm, light wind and note how the leaves of the trees sway in the breeze.
- Heighten your gaze and note the clear, blue sky.
- Lower your gaze and observe the beds of flowers and rose bushes in the foreground.
- Imagine yourself now rising from your chair and walking over to the pink rosebush. Note how it is abundantly filled with roses at all stages of development. Look at the buds, the flowers in full bloom, and those that are fading. Look at the petals all over the ground at the base of the bush.
- Focus on a mature rose in full bloom. Look carefully at the flower and lean over to smell it.
- Inhale the scent of rose perfume that permeates the air surrounding the bush. Breathe deeply and enjoy the rich, fragrant odor.
- Note the perfection of the flower. Feel its velvet petals and once more inhale its perfuse, lovely smell.
- Thank the rose for offering you its gift and then return to settle in your chair in the center of the garden.
- Feel the peace and serenity of this special place. Realize that you can return to this place whenever you desire. You need only to quiet your thoughts and relax your body-mind.
- Say good-bye to your special place and return your attention to the present. Focus again on the here and now.

Observations

Did you enjoy this exercise? Did you feel that you were actually in a garden? Did you smell the roses? The power of imagery is so great that our senses can interpret visual pictures as actually occuring.

If you, or the client you guide, do not have immediate results, or do not see the pictures or have other sensory sensations, do not despair. The development of this skill, like any other, takes time and practice. People perceive in various ways; some are visual while others are auditory, tactile, or olfactory. It may take longer for some to develop this perceptual and actualizing skill. Try another exercise now.

Your Healthy Body

- Once again position yourself in a comfortable place. Allow yourself to take several deep breaths. Continue with the progressive relaxation technique until you feel your body completely supported and comfortable in your chair.
- Imagine yourself standing up and walking toward a full-length mirror. Look at the reflection you see before you. As you do this, imagine the figure you see before you is the healthy, happy person that you would like to become. Note the silhouette and see the definitions in body torso. Observe your posture straight and upright. See your skin as healthy and glowing and your hair shiny and clean.
- Begin to move as you observe the reflection in the mirror. Fully extend your limbs and feel your body becoming supple and strong.
- Sense that your internal organs are firm and fully functioning. Feel the power of your invigorated, healthy body.
- Realize that this is the way you want to look and feel.
  This is the healthy you that you are creating by eating, moving, and thinking well and applying the self-discipline you have within yourself.
- Look one last time at this healthy figure and know that you create your own reality. The person you are seeing in the reflection is your healthy self.
- Bid farewell to this image and return your focus to the present.

Each time we use self-talk or imagery we need to focus the picture or words in the present tense. For example, in this healthy-self exercise, your attention is directed to see the image as if it already existed. We have learned from science that our brain creates what it believes. Consequently, if the image we give it is what we want to become, then circumstances will occur that allow that image to manifest. When one works with visualization in earnest, then other aspects of the self begin to operationalize to create the desired reality. If you practice this exercise repeatedly, you will more than likely begin to exercise, eat properly, focus on good posture, and take better care of yourself in general. Since we are holistic beings, whenever we change one aspect of ourselves, all other parts change too.

Imagery Techniques

For best results when using imagery remember the following:
- Be clear about your desired outcome.
- Focus on visualizing as many details about the situation as possible.
- Mentally walk through the entire script focusing on the events or action you want to happen.
- Visualize the best possible scenario.
- Use imagery to prepare for positive outcomes of upcoming events. See yourself as successful.

USING IMAGERY WITH CLIENTS

The nurse healer will find ample opportunities to guide clients through the imagery process. Almost any client situation will respond to the use of imagery. The nurse healer must first ascertain what and how much the client knows about this technique. Before using guided imagery first ask the clients if they desire this therapy. Often it is necessary to explain what it is and how it works. Many clients may be hesitant or afraid to develop fantasy scenarios. Steps to assist another in this process are as follows:

1. Ask the clients to get into a comfortable position. If at all possible, have them recline and close their eyes.

2. Guide the clients in deep breathing and use progressive-relaxation suggestions.

3. Begin suggesting relaxing and peaceful images.

4. Continue to guide them to focus on their breathing, physical relaxation, and images of a safe, secure setting.

5. Have the clients focus on the issue at hand (e.g., wound healing, combating infection).

6. Guide the clients to see a positive resolution of their problem or issue of concern.

7. Ask the clients to verbalize what they are seeing or feeling.

8. Guide the clients to close their fantasy scenario and, when they are ready, to open their eyes and return their focus to the here and now.

9. Talk with the clients about the meaning and significance of what occurred during the imagery event.

10. Guide the clients to verbalize insights gleaned from the imagery. Reinforce the positive aspects of manifesting a healing reality.

When clients realize that you are there to assist them with a noninvasive, self-healing process, this usually allays their fear of the unknown. When they are in a trusting, relaxed state, they will be more open to trying a new technique. After an initial exposure that maintains their sense of security and being in control of the situation, clients generally become open to being guided with this modality. Suggestions for use of imagery in the clinical area include the following:

Acute Care Settings

- Perioperative area—successful surgical procedures
- Postoperative areas—swift recovery and surgical site healing
- Burn units—wound healing, skin grafting
- Orthopedic units—bone grafting
- Cardiac units—artery reanastomosis, developing collateral circulation
- Oncology—successful results of chemotherapy or radiation
- Obstetrics—facilitating the delivery process, involuting the reproductive organs following birth, or beginning successful infant lactation
- Pediatrics—guiding the child to visualize a successful outcome of the specific therapy

Health Promotion, Wellness, and Stress Management

In this arena of care nurse healers can successfully use imagery in many areas. Some of these are as follows:

- Stress management, conflict resolution, time management
- Life-style behavior modification
- Preparation for new skill development
- Working through relationship problems
- Improving communication skills
- Maximizing creative potential
- Imaging a steady state of high level wellness
- Opening to the full human potential

These ideas represent just a few ways that imagery can be used. Guiding with imagery can be a powerful tool for the nurse healer.

Healer Reflections

How did I feel when following the imagery exercise in this chapter?

Can I see in colors, perceive shapes and forms, and feel tactile sensations?

Did I smell the roses in the exercise?

In what setting might I use guided imagery with clients?

What could I do to feel comfortable using imagery with clients?

Do I value this skill?

Chapter 16

Music

Music is the mediator between the spirit and the sensual life.

Ludwig van Beethoven (1770–1827)

Empowering Yourself

Realize that music has been used in healing since antiquity.

Understand that all living organisms emit and receive sensations through vibrations, sound, and rhythm.

Know that music is believed to be the most powerful of all the art forms.

Discover how healing can occur with music therapy.

RHYTHM AND VIBRATION

The entire animal kingdom is conditioned to vibration, sound, and rhythm. In nonhuman species of life we have recorded delicate, vibrational sensitivities. Fish, for example, have a "lateral line" organ that runs the whole length of their bodies from head to tail. This line registers water pressure and receives vibrations or sounds that we can now detect with sensitive electronic devices. Many species of insects and birds turn their body parts into "musical instruments." Some creatures have highly evolved their music as they communicate with one another. The singing of birds is reflected in the tones discernible in the flute, trumpet, violin, and drum. Humans live in a world of vibrations that, although we have refined and turned to our advantage, we are still exploring. Next to the eye, the ear is our most valuable sense. Sound waves intersect our brains to literally convert matter into mind. It is from vibrations and rhythm that our brain converts messages to neural impulses, to sensations, to feelings, to emotions, and then into aesthetic, spiritual, social, and healing meanings.

MUSIC AS AN ART

The arts have always served as a medium for bringing people together and uniting them. Art forms penetrate our senses to arouse emotions, stir the intellect, and even cause physiologic body changes, and of all the arts, music is perhaps the most compelling. Carefully selected music has the capacity to create unity in even the most heterogeneous mix of people and to promote calm in the most chaotic of situations.

Music is pleasurable because it is one of the few arts that helps to relieve stress and tension. Music has long been used to help sublimate aggressive and destructive behavior. Sublimation is easier with the help of music because listening to music offers more opportunity than any other art for muscular action and motion. Music's rhythm, which stimulates body rhythm, gives us an opportunity to feel ourselves not only more integrated and organized but also capable of easy and graceful physical expression. We associate words, sounds, and musical symbols with pleasant or disagreeable emotional memories.

MUSIC AS THERAPY

Words Versus Music

Psychotherapy is the utilization of words, their meanings, and the dynamics behind them for the purpose of changing behavior. The meanings of words appeal primarily to the cerebral hemisphere, the master brain. After they pass through the cerebral hemisphere, emotional reactions and organ functions follow. Verbal therapy has long been recognized by healers, philosophers, writers, poets, preachers, and teachers.

In contrast to verbal therapy, music therapy lends itself to healing because it meets with little or no intellectual resistance and does not need to appeal to logic or analysis. It is more subtle and more primitive, and therefore its appeal is wider and greater. Music touches the unconscious aspect of our being and can arouse responses that no verbal therapy can induce.

APPLICATION IN CLINICAL SETTINGS

The potential value in healing with music is profound. Music is capable of changing moods by stirring the listener to overcome depressed feelings, to calm overactive activity, to find release through an instinctual behavior, and to be inspired to go on in the face of obstacles. Since music has this power, it is important to recognize its application in appropriate clinical settings with clients.

Psychotherapy

Using music in health promotion, psychotherapy, or guided one-on-one sessions can promote healing in remarkable ways.

Laura's Story

Laura, a 30-year-old, single, elementary-school teacher, was referred to a nurse psychotherapist when medical practitioners were unable to diagnose or help her. Her symptoms included longstanding dysmenorrhea, tightness and pain on both sides of the neck, and pains in the face and head. When she came for therapy she was on a leave of absence from work. She was worn out with worry, indecisive, self-centered, and preoccupied. She spent hours daydreaming and watching herself in the mirror and was conscious of a lump and a metallic taste in her throat.

Appointments were scheduled for the nurse to begin intensive therapy with her three to four times a week. During the initial visits a strong musical background was revealed. Before entering college she use to sing and play the piano "by ear." The nurse decided to try music therapy as the healing modality. An expert music teacher was secured for vocal lessons. In addition, the nurse advised Laura to move out of her parents' house into an apartment with two other working women her own age.

The first stage of her therapy involved thrice weekly voice lessons where she was instructed to exercise and rest each day in addition to practicing her music. Her voice teacher taught her relaxation exercises of the throat, mouth, and body muscles and the art of tone and breathing. Both the nurse and the music teacher initially found her extremely tense and stiff.

It took Laura 7 weeks of daily exercise to finally relax the neck, throat, and jaw muscles and to produce a free and open tone. She claimed that each new exercise caused tenseness and pain, but by conscious effort she learned to develop confidence in relaxing before singing. When she relapsed into pain and quivers she was told to stop, relax, and begin again. By the end of 2 months she was able to relax her jaw completely and produce the high C with ease.

After a vacation of 3 weeks the second period of therapy began. This time she progressed quickly, and at the end of the second month both she and the nurse therapist declared her healed. Laura described herself as "growing happy from the inside out." She said, "I am beginning to manage and direct myself instead of allowing a stampede of forces to control me. I am alive with ambition." Laura changed her path from wandering pitifully around the house with hot water bottles on her pains to a direction that incorporated her renewed love for music with her elementary teaching. She moved to a rural area and became the seventh grade teacher in a small school. She included song, rhythm, and instruments in all aspects of her teaching. Two years later she was recognized for innovative excellence in teaching. Without music therapy Laura may have continued to suffer and society would have not have benefited from her contributions.

Acute Care

Music audiocassettes can be used in the acute-care area to soothe or distract patients. Settings for the use of personal headsets for music cassettes are multiple and include the following:

- Perioperative holding areas
- Cardiac care units
- Rehabilitation
- Sleep induction

Classification of Music

Therapeutic music generally lulls and relaxes. Discordant, loud music should be avoided since it agitates and excites.

The particular type of music you should select will depend on the client's personal preference and the goals of the therapy. Therapeutic music can be classified as follows:

1. Mood music—slow, fast

2. Classical music—slow, fast

3. Romantic music—slow, fast

4. Impressionist music—slow, fast

5. Rock and roll music—soft

6. Country music

7. New age music

When a nurse healer uses music with clients the following benefits can occur:

1. Changes in metabolism and endocrine activity

2. Lowering of respiration, blood pressure, pulse, and muscular-energy activity

3. Improvement in attention span

4. Distraction and diversion

5. Opportunity to replace negative emotions with new uplifting feelings and ideas

6. Stimulation of the capacity to visualize and image

Healer Reflections

What kind of music soothes and relaxes me?

Can I remember a time when I used music to help me through a difficult situation?

How do I feel about using music as a healing modality?

In what setting could I use music with my clients?

Do I believe in the power of music to heal?

Chapter 17

Meditation and Prayer

Empowering Yourself

Understand that meditation has been used as a tool for mental development and discipline for millennia.

Be aware that effective meditation requires consistent practice.

Know that routine use of effective meditation can strengthen your ability to solve problems.

Realize that prayer has been acknowledged as a source of comfort, healing, and miraculous cures since antiquity.

MEDITATION

Meditation is a technique used to quiet the mind. It involves the conscious focus of attention on an object, breathing technique, mantra, mandala, or mental picture to achieve a mental goal. Most of those who believe the technique will work for them and follow through with the discipline necessary to learn the art have both physiological and psychological responses. When the body-mind undergoes deep relaxation that is possible in a meditative state, the autonomic nervous system responds with a decrease in heart rate, lower blood pressure, decreased respiratory rate and oxygen consumption, changes in electroencephalogram activity, and a lower arousal threshold. When meditation is practiced over a period, meditators report psychological calming and a sense of control over their emotions.

Meditation is an ancient art practiced extensively in Hindu, Taoist, and Buddhist antiquity, as well as in the more recent Judeo-Christian tradition. All cultures and religions have practiced and still do practice some form of meditation.

Why Meditate?

There are as many answers to this question as there are people to ask it. Many meditate to achieve the following:
- Decrease stress
- Access more of their human potential
- Build zest and enthusiasm for life
- Find or recover lost parts of the self
- Increase awareness of our unity with the universe
- Improve ability to see and function in day-to-day reality more effectively
- Strengthen their spiritual connection
- Increase stamina
- Quiet and discipline the mind

Nurse healers use meditation for all of the above reasons in addition to others of their own. Once the modality is mastered by the practitioner, it is an excellent tool for use in multiple practice settings. Some areas in which meditation has been effectively employed include the following:
- Rehabilitation
- Stress management
- Cardiac care units

- Life-style behavioral counseling
- Health and wellness promotion

Meditation Techniques

Practioners of this skill will hasten their ability to meditate if they first master the skills of breathing, progressive relaxation, and imagery. Meditation is the next step in this series of therapies. A variety of techniques ranging from individual contemplation to group circles to unstructured techniques are available to induce the state of meditation. Once the specific form is chosen the meditator progresses along the following steps:

1. Find a quiet, comfortable place to sit.

2. With your back straight and palms supported on your thighs, close your eyes.

3. Follow the deep-breathing and/or progressive-relaxation exercises.

4. Focus on the mental image of choice and concentrate on it single-mindedly. This focus will vary from person to person. It may be on nostril flaring, a picture mandala, a spoken mantra, or a specific mental image. Allow distracting thoughts that drift into your mind to gently float out without giving them your attention.

5. When you have achieved your goal, open your eyes and come back to the present.

It is suggested that this process be practiced on a daily basis for 10 to 15 minutes. Following the meditation some people find it beneficial to write in a journal. Recording and analyzing the process over time reaps additional benefits.

PRAYER

If you should never see my face again,
Pray for my soul. More things are wrought by prayer
Than this world dreams of. Wherefore, let your voice
Rise like a fountain for me night and day.
For what are people better than sheep or goats
That nourish a blind life within the brain,
If knowing God, they lift not hands of prayer

Both for themselves and those who call them friend?

For so the whole round earth is every way

Bound by gold chains about the feet of God.

Alfred, Lord Tennyson (1809–1892)

Prayer differs from meditation in that it usually involves direct application to God, a saint, or some person to intervene directly between the one who prays and the one who answers the prayer. Prayer, like meditation, is a part of our ancestral heritage and has been used throughout recorded history. It is an important part of many nurse healers' skill repertoire. In prayer we are told to ask, seek, and knock and that the door will be open to us. Prayer is said to be the key to unlock the door to spiritual blessings.

Penny's Story

During the spring of her last semester in nursing school Penny gave birth to her second child. Despite being weakened by a month of flu and pneumonia during the Christmas holiday, she returned to school and continued to fully prepare for all her class assignments and even help others as a tutor. Her labor started during the first day of spring break. She endured a grueling, 20-hour labor with inadequate cervical dilation. The baby was eventually delivered by cesarean section.

Penny returned to classes after spring break with her nursing infant. During her first 2 weeks back after break, the faculty arranged alternative clinical assignments for her that involved library work and oral reports to the post-conference group. She was determined to succeed with her studies and to give the best possible care to her new infant. The faculty arranged a time and place that Penny's mother could bring in the new baby during the course of the biweekly 7-hour clinical shift so that she could nurse the baby. She was a student who was cheerful and well liked and who worked diligently to succeed. In May she graduated at the top of her class with high honors.

Ten months later Penny was diagnosed with breast cancer. She underwent mastectomy followed by chemotherapy and radiation. Since she had always followed a healthy life-style, she was confused and unclear about why she had to face this consequence. Despite her optimistic efforts and compliance with the medical regime, her condition continued to deteriorate. She developed a secondary infection and was told she might die. It was at this point that her once abiding faith in God turned to anger. How could He let her down, she had prayed so hard, she had done everything right, she had believed her prayers would work, and here she was dying.

Since Penny had returned for periodic visits with the faculty after graduation, they stayed connected with her. It was at this point that one of the faculty became intimately involved. She went from a hospital visit with Penny directly to her Wednesday night prayer group. She passionately told them Penny's story. On hearing the tragic details of this young woman's life, they initiated an intense group prayer effort. Led by the faculty member they were able to visualize all the details of Penny's life and circumstances. They fervently prayed for her full recovery. Remarkably Penny began to have a medical turnaround. Week after week the group continued to pray for this physically unseen but spiritually present person. The faculty prayer group member continued to paint specific visual images for the group as they steadfastly prayed for Penny. Within a short time Penny's prognosis changed from terminal, to guarded, to serious, . . . to recovery. Penny overcame the infection, began to respond to radiation, and within 8 months' time was pronounced cured.

During a cold, Sunday morning in January, 1 year after initial diagnosis, Penny, her husband, and their two small children traveled to the faculty members' church to give personal testimony. No one but the faculty member and the pastor had ever actually seen her physically, but as she stood at the pulpit giving a compelling testimony to the power of prayer and the miracle it had caused in her life, she awakened the hearts of everyone present. There were no dry eyes as she linked her path of recovery to several prayer groups, which she believed made the difference between her present life and her possible death. Today Penny practices nursing in an emergency room and quietly uses prayer as one of her personal favorite nursing interventions. She knows its power.

Healer Reflections

Am I open to trying to meditate?

What changes have I witnessed in my own body as I sit for meditation?

Am I willing to set aside 10 to 15 minutes each day to practice this skill?

When was the last time I became involved with prayer?

Do I believe that miracles can happen with prayer?

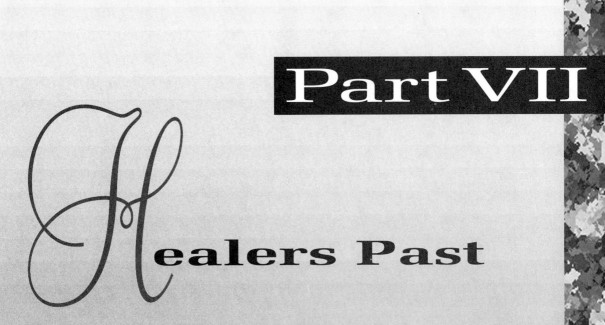

Part VII

Healers Past and Present: Our Ancestral Heritage

Spirit and Magic: Healers in Antiquity

The natural healing force within each one of us is the greatest force in getting well.

Hippocrates

Empowering Yourself

Become aware of the origin of the spirit-healer connection?

What is your connection with spirit?

Become aware of what symbols you use in your healing practice.

Become aware of mythological symbolism in the collective unconscious.

Become aware of the differences between how the Greeks and Romans used water for healing.

SPIRIT AND MAGIC

From the dawn of humankind people have been fascinated by the healing process. From the earliest times healers have used their creative forces to explore and utilize everything that their time and culture afforded them to augment the ever mysterious healing process.

Healing in ancient, tribal cultures was rich with color and form and filled with spirit. It was replete with ritual, ceremony, magic, and drama. In many instances healing sites and rituals were as important as the actual healer interventions. This was the dawn of the era of spirit and magic. Healing was a revered art, and the healers themselves were believed to have a direct link with the gods. They were the sacred practitioners.

Early tribal peoples were closely aligned with the earth and natural law and had an ongoing relationship with the animal and plant kingdoms. Early people believed all natural objects—rocks, rivers, trees, wind, and animals—were alive and possessed a spirit or soul. They had a belief in the interconnectedness of all things as integral to the healing ritual. This belief had a profound effect on the development of practices for the treatment of maladies.

In antiquity it was believed that many illnesses were the result of spiritual imbalance, so many cures were attempted through activation of the spiritual domain. Consequently, a great body of tribal lore developed that included incantations, rites, rituals, and spells. The primary goal was to manipulate the body in such a fashion that it would be an unpleasant place for evil spirits and thus the body would be rid of the cause of the illness.

As this magical lore accumulated, it became too complex to be easily understood by the ordinary tribespeople, so individuals with special insight were selected to devote their time to mastering and interpreting the spiritual realms to the others. The possession of life-giving powers granted these "medicine men and women" or "shamans" a place of prestige and set them apart from the ordinary person. Thus the esoteric position of the healer and the devotion to the pursuit of the alleviation of pain and suffering began.

THE SHAMAN

The word shaman was originally derived from the Sanskrit **sramana**, meaning to exhaust or fatigue. This is perhaps in reference to the exhausting, epileptic-type seizures that the healers exhibited when working their magic. In English usage, shaman comes from a Greek modification of the Russian modification of the Tungusic **saman,** which derives from the Pali **samana**, 'a Buddhist monk,' which comes from the Sanskrit word.

Jeanne Achterberg (1985) describes the shaman's role in the history of healing. In prehistoric times the shaman was the artist, dancer, poet, clown, and healer and was often gifted in most of the entertainment arts. The shaman could relate to guardian spirits from whom power and knowledge was gained. Thus the shaman, as well as being a healer, served and still serves in some areas of the world such as Sri Lanka and New Guinea as a philosopher/priest with access to supernatural reality.

Shamanic practice involves the use of these talents to move in and out of special states of consciousness with the purpose of helping others. Unlike some other mystics, shamans do not seek enlightenment for its sake alone, but for the specific purpose of healing or in some manner aiding the community. They follow a circular path moving in and out of other realms of consciousness, returning each time with new knowledge and power for use in healing.

HEALERS IN CLASSICAL TIMES

All cultures and civilizations played a significant role in the evolution of contemporary healing. Our ancestors in the Western tradition included healers from ancient Egypt, Babylonia, Assyria, Palestine, India, Persia, Greece, Rome, and the Celtic world. The striking quality of all noted healers from antiquity was the close relationship of the healer to a god, goddess, or grouping of deities. Mythology is rich with legends linking gods and mortals. The first recorded documents were from ancient Egypt. It is in these, and the subsequent recordings of other early civilizations, that we see the evolution of the healers' direct connection with god (the shaman) emerge into the role of priest/priestess-healer.

THE EGYPTIANS (4000—600 B.C.)

Egypt was the first civilization to emerge into the light of wisdom. These ancients were a people of superior attainments, the highest achievers becoming the priest/priestess-healers. They were both male and female, highly educated, and famed throughout the Orient from earliest times.

Both the Egyptians and the Babylonions believed that sickness resulted from the demonic ill will of various gods or evil spirits. The dualistic Persians thought of disease as one activity of the powers of darkness. Healing in these cultures embodied the techniques of expelling the ill will of the gods or the demons themselves.

THE GREEKS (700 B.C.–300 A.D.)

Greek culture offers perhaps the most colorful and interesting array of healers. The Greek ideal was to achieve balance in all aspects of living and to have a sound mind housed within a strong body. In the world of ancient Greece, many institutions dedicated to healing arose. There were over 200 temples called Asclepions, named after Asclepius, the God of healing. These centers, which existed for approximately 1000 years, were complete with mythology, symbolism, and priest/priestess healers who utilized a method of healing that incorporated all the knowledge of the era. When an ailing person sought healing, total immersion in a physical, mental, and spiritual healing environment ensued. Dreams, drama, music, art, laughter, massage, bathing, and rest were used along with herbs and the basic surgical treatments available.

Hygeia was renown as a feminine healer. From her name the term hygiene, meaning sanitary cleanliness, was derived. It was thought that initially she had no special relationship to the demigod Asclepius, but when she arrived at the temple in Epidaurus and began to do healing work, she came to be regarded as his daughter. Some legends say she was his wife, while others state she eventually assimilated with him and lost an independent personality. Whatever the case, there was identification with him. Hygieia, as well as her sister Panacea, represented the importance of the feminine aspect of the healing arts. Her influence was so great that the cult of Hygieia spread alongside Asclepius and was introduced into the Roman Empire in 293 B.C. During the period of classical Greek mythology Asclepius and Hygeia were recognized as the god and goddess of healing.

Hippocrates is perhaps the best known of all healers from antiquity, the father of Western medicine. According to legend, Hippocrates was born on the island of Cos, part of the Greek island chain, around 460 B.C. As a young man he traveled to the famous temple of Asclepius and studied the knowledge and practices of Asclepiadaes (the priest/priestess-physicians) handed down through oral tradition from the demigod Asclepius. The characteristic that made Hippocrates unique was that he prolifically translated these oral traditions and knowledge into written form. By 500 B.C. Hippocrates had cataloged and written about many methods of scientific treatment. The 57 volumes that survived the centuries are divided into many of the same subspeciality categories that we use today.

During this era medicine was practiced without any reference to nursing. However, because formal nursing developed around the same logical, organizational content, this material involving the evolution and development of medicine is included here.

Hippocrates and his team symbolized the change in the practice of medicine from the mystical/mythological to the use of natural/logical principles. He believed, like Florence Nightingale who followed centuries later, that the healer's role was to understand and assist nature in allowing the body to heal itself. He felt it was important to know a person's relationship to food, drink, and occupation because they affected health and illness. He, like Asclepius before him, espoused the healing qualities of gentleness, concern, love, and dignity.

Plato recognized the prime need for curing the soul to find real healing of the body. He saw healing as one of the ways in which Divine creative energy comes to possess human beings. Throughout his writings he stresses the necessity of curing disease by treating the whole person. In his book *Phaedrus* he lists healing along with prophecy, art, and love as a way in which he saw the Divine breaking through and manifesting itself in the physical world. Although Plato embraced the healing that occurred in the temples of Aesculapius, the basic understanding of this concept reached fruition in the early Christian churches.

Aristotle, a comtemporary of Plato, rejected the concept of divine healing because he rejected any elementary principle of evil in the world.

By the close of the Greek era the acknowledgment and use of spirit in healing was at its height. The beginning of scientific inquiry would advance and poliferate as new civilizations blossomed.

THE ROMAN PERIOD (750 B.C.—400 A.D.)

One healing tradition blended into another as the Greek Empire declined and the Roman Empire emerged and expanded. Throughout the literature of Greece and Rome, ideas are expressed that sick people were suffering from the displeasure of the gods. The same god that brought disease could also bring healing.

One of the health benefits of being a Roman citizen was the use of therapeutic baths. The healing sites in Greece were always located by water, but it was the Romans who expanded this concept and developed health spas. For example, the baths of Diocletian (245–313 A.D.) contained 3000 rooms. When patrons came for therapy they first entered the Apodyterium, where they were undressed and massaged. Then they went to the Tepidarium, which was warm and balmy, followed by the warm Sudatorium, which produced marked sweating, then into the hot bath, the Calidarium, and finally into the cold bath, the Frigidarium. By the time of Emperor Constantine toward the end of the Empire, there were 860 baths and 11 large thermae in Rome.

The effect of the baths in early Roman history was not simply cleansing of the body but a ritualistic cleansing of mind and spirit as the body was washed. However, by the later Roman periods the Hellenistic influence of the spiritual connotation of the baths had been all but abandoned.

THE CELTS

The Celtic tradition spanned innumerable centuries. Some speculate that the Celts lived as long ago as the Egyptians and that elements of the culture still exist today in the contemporary world. Originally they lived throughout the continent of Europe but were eventually pushed to the outer limits of France, Scotland, Wales, and Ireland.

LINKAGE OF THE ANCIENT WORLD WITH MODERN HEALING

The understanding of the linkage of the ancient Graeco-Roman world with modern healing can be understood in the attitudes of the early Christians who were the residents of that world. Their leader, Jesus Christ, broke radically with both the Judaic heritage and with the Greaco-Roman world. Many authors and Biblical critics see the Christians' mission embodied in his life, acts, teaching, and practice as a return to a shamanism based on an intimate relationship with a loving Father. He became a mediator between a person's body and their spiritual reality, a healer of body, mind, and spirit. The Christians' message was that the power of God had broken through into our world and that evil has been put to flight. Jesus saw himself as the Messiah representing the essential nature of God himself, acting as his messenger. His healings therefore were rooted in the essential nature of God. The Graeco-Roman inhabitants of his world rapidly embraced his philosophy and psychology, and the Asclepiads became the Christian shrines.

The early Christians believed that people had conscious control not only of their personalities but also of their destinies. The skills to produce change only needed to be exercised and developed. The mark of the early Christian society was "conscious control." The powerful impact of this concept to change the existing social order led to the persecution of the Christians by the Roman state.

THE EASTERN WORLD

At the same time healers emerged in the West similar events were unfolding in Asia. Dhanvantari of India, like Asclepius of Greece, was a mythological physician of the gods. He is said to have emerged from the churning of the ocean by the gods bearing the cup of amrita or the nectar of immortality.

India: Ayurvedic Medicine

Dhanvantari was the founder of Ayurveda, Sanskrit for "the science of life." Ayurveda has a preventive, holistic focus and has been practiced in India for over 4000 years. It is believed to be the parent of Oriental medicine as well as Greek medicine. Ayurveda is concerned with eight principal branches of medicine. In this system each ailment is addressed according to theories of the five elements (ether, air, fire, water, and earth), the three bodily humors, the body tissues, the body excretions, and the trinity of life (body, mind, and spiritual awareness).

Healing from the Ayurvedic perspective was primarily concerned with the inward search and the quest for spiritual growth. The theory of reincarnation affected every aspect of life, including the treatment of illness and the acceptance of death.

A related system to Ayureveda is yoga. Yoga is a means of psychophysiological self-regulation aimed at longevity, rejuvenation, and self-realization. Practiced in a variety of forms, yoga is performed to speed up the natural evolution of the individual. Yoga deals with the unfoldment of human consciousness with the purpose of eventually reaching total enlightenment. It was believed that when left on his own without the discipline of yoga, man would more slowly evolve through the inevitable suffering that is a condition of earthly life.

It was through the Indian healing system that Western people gained knowledge of chakras. Chakras are unseen energy fields consisting of vortices of energy that can be activated by concentration or meditation. It is believed that the chakras, like the Chinese meridians, can become stagnant or blocked, hence giving rise to illness. There are seven major chakras located along the anterior body from the top of the head to the base of the spinal column. In contrast to Western healers who tended to do something to someone else to alleviate sickness, the Vedic system teaches activation of the chakra energy centers for self-healing. However, they too had knowledge of herbs and roots and an early understanding of anatomy and physiology.

The Orient

Healers in China and Japan developed a different system with the focus on the movement of life energy (ch'i) along a system of unseen, internal pathways called meridians. It is on these meridians that the acupuncture and acupressure points are located. The flow of ch'i is affected by balance of the opposing energies called yin and yang. The yin and yang are fundamentally female and male polar energies with many attributes accorded to each. It is believed that when the balance between yin and yang is disturbed, illness or dis-ease occurs. One of the treatments for illness in this system is the insertion of acupuncture needles in one or more of the hundreds of points along the meridians for the purpose of stimulating and restoring the flow of the ch'i energy.

The development of medicine in the Orient was based on the following applied theories: orbisiconography (functional relationships within the body), sinarteriology, (the natural channeling of ch'i energy through meridians of the body), pharmaceutical agents, change in climatic environment, and immunology. The sciences of organic anatomy, histology, and biochemistry were not developed because they did not fit into their theoretical framework of healing. The Chinese treated illness according to how energy flowed in relation to the energy of the universe.

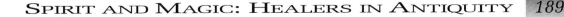

Summary

Since antiquity various individuals and healing systems have played a valuable role in awakening the evolving elements that have followed. The modern nurse healer can draw on one million years of human, unconscious evolution to learn the intuitive processes of the past and to then add to those the scientific processes of the present to consciously create the healing synthesis of the future.

Healer Reflections

How would it feel to adorn my clothing with symbolic ornaments and allow myself to enter a trancelike state as I call on the spirits to work through me as I practice healing today?

Are there any deities from antiquity that have special meaning in my life today?

If I were a shaman, what would go on in my mind and how would I channel healing from the universe of animism?

How would I feel as a patron in one of the great healing spas at the height of the Roman Empire?

REFERENCES

Achterberg, J. *Imagery in healing.* Boston: New Science Library, 1985.

Berman, M. *The reenchantment of the world.* Ithaca, N.Y.: Cornell University Press, 1981.

Jayne, W. A. *The healing god of ancient civilization.* New York: University Books, 1962.

Lad, V. *Ayurveda: The science of self-healing.* Santa Fe, Calif.: Lotus Press, 1985.

Lyons, A. S. & Petrucelli, R. J., II *Medicine: An illustrated history.* New York: Abradale Press, 1987.

Sanford, J. A. *Healing and wholeness.* New York: Paulist Press, 1977.

Thomson, W. A. *Spas that heal.* London: Adam and Charles Black, 1978.

The Age of Faith:
Medieval Years

Thy faith hath made thee whole.

St. Matthew

Empowering Yourself

Observe that different cultures within the same time period practiced different modes of healing.

Consider what qualities one had to possess to emerge as a healer during this era.

Be aware of the continuing link of the priest/priestess healer and the shaman.

Recognize that sometimes healing abilities come to us through illuminations, visions, or imagery.

THE RISE OF CHRISTIANITY

Toward the end of the Roman Empire there began to be noticeable flaws in the social order of the system. The minority became rich and powerful, while the masses were either poverty-stricken or indentured servants. The value of life was lessened by demonstrations such as public coliseum events featuring Christians being thrown to the lions. Exhaustion of supplies, corruption, and general dissatisfaction led to the fall of the empire and the development of the age of faith.

During a period of change and confusion, Christianity dominated the European continent. As we have seen in the previous chapter, this religion was based on the teachings of Jesus Christ and was spread throughout the region by his apostles and disciples. The concept of one loving God of all humanity was good news to the poor, sick, and needy of the day. The decisive act that ushered in the new religion was taken by the Roman Emperor Constantine. In 313 A.D. he had a vision of a burning cross in the sky that said, "In this sign you will conquer." Following this vision he fought and won a decisive battle and proclaimed freedom for the church. From this point forward the Christianization of the Roman Empire began.

To many the next thousand years were seen as dreary and gloomy. Some historians call this period "the dark ages"; however, in restrospect we can call it "the age of faith." For it was faith in something greater than oneself, faith for endurance during difficult times, and faith in the future that perpetuated the survival of the human race for many generations to come.

THE AGE OF FAITH
(800 A.D.–1600 A.D.)

During the age of faith, Christianity was the glue that held the Western world together. Unlike the pagan religions, which tended to abandon people thought to have incurred the disfavor of the gods, the Christian church emphasized the need for reenactment of Christ's healing mission. It was not the healer but the Grace of God that provided a cure. Hence, in the Western world those who took on the attitudes and behaviors of Christ were the ones who emerged as healers. Many of them assumed the humility of Christ and allowed his healing source to pass through them as a conduit.

During the unchallenged expansion of the Catholic church, the bishops emerged as the self-appointed leaders of the people. It was this

Christianization of the land that contributed to the evolution of the image of the nurse as a saint. The activity of nursing became honored as many royal, noble, and distinguished people turned to nursing, regarding it as the work of God. It also became the penitential activity used as a means of purgation and purification. Nursing was work of unceasing toil undertaken with no expectation of earthly reward.

Fabiola was a Roman matron. Having been unhappily married twice, following the death of her second husband, she converted to Christianity, renounced her earthly pleasures, and became a nun. She used her immense fortune to establish the first free Christian hospital in Rome in 390 A.D. Fabiola sought out the sick and poor in the streets of Rome and cared for them herself. It is said that she became particularly skilled with the most ugly and repugnant wounds and sores. She is revered as one of the early patron saints of nursing (Donahue, 1985). A famous eulogy by St. Jerome given in 399 A.D. depicts her life:

> There she gathered together all the sick from the highways and streets, and herself nursed the unhappy, emaciated victims of hunger and disease. Can I describe here the varied scourges which afflict human beings?—the mutilated, blinded countenances, the partially destroyed limbs, the livid hands, swollen bodies, and wasted extremities? . . . How often have I seen her carrying in her arms these piteous, dirty, and revolting victims of a frightful malady! How often have I seen her wash wounds whose fetid odour prevented every one else from even looking at them! She fed the sick with her own hands, and revived the dying with small and frequent portions of nourishment. I know that many wealthy persons cannot overcome the repugnance caused by such works of charity; . . . I do not judge them, . . . but if I had a hundred tongues and a clarion voice I could not enumerate the number of patients for whom Fabiola provided solace and care. The poor who were well envied those who were sick.

> *St. Jerome, Letter to Oceanus*

Monasticism

During the 1000-year period from 476 to 1453 A.D. the Germanic Huns invaded all of what we know today as Europe. They destroyed all the great libraries, works of art, theatres, and shrines, including all culture that had been developed up to this time. The last of the Roman emperors fled to Constantinople as the empire was overrun by barbarians and collapsed in 476 A.D.

It was at this time that orders of monks and nuns emerged, banding together to form the first cloistered communities. Here in monasteries and convents dedicated men and women cared for the sick and diseased and preserved the knowledge of the ancient world. These orders were made up of both men and women who, based on the concept of Christian charity and its imagery of the presence of the spirit in the body of man, made a virtue of what were called the corporal works of mercy. These works of mercy nourished the spirit of both the caregiver and those receiving the care. The orientation of the healers during this 1000-year period was totally holistic; it incorporated into every healing process an interlinking of body, mind, and spirit even to the point of considering some diseases as caused by the presence of evil spirits and treating these maladies by exorcism.

VISION AND ILLUMINATIONS

Hildegard of Bingen (1098–1179) was the youngest of ten children in a German family attached to the Castle of Bickelheim on the Rhine river in the town of Bingen. Hildegard was educated by a tutor from the Benedictine monastery in the traditions of music, Bible history, spinning, prayer, and work. At the age of 18 she joined the monastery (in those days, men and women shared the same community). When Hildegard was 38 her predecessor died, and she took over the leadership of the female community. It was 4 years later when she had her spiritual awakening. She told us, "When I was forty-two and seven months old, a burning light of tremendous brightness coming from heaven poured into my entire mind. Like a flame that does not burn but enkindles, it inflamed my entire heart and my entire breast, just like the sun that warms an object with its rays. All of a sudden, I was able to taste of the understanding of the narration of books." Overcome by this experience of intuition, connection-making, and insight, she retired to a sickbed. Following another illumination, when she placed her hand to writing, she recovered her strength and got out of bed. She spent the next 10 years writing her first book.

Her written illuminations consisted of text and paintings to encourage the divine flow from human hearts. Like the light of the sun, her heart was inflamed, and she felt the need to awaken other hearts so that imagination, creativity, forgiveness, and contrition might flow again in the world. She told people to "wake up, take responsibility, and make choices." In her book *Scivias* she advises readers to "know the ways," meaning know the wise ways as distinct from the foolish ways. She believed that people who follow the ways of wisdom "will themselves become a fountain gushing from the waters of life." Among her many contributions she continually extolled the virtue of "usefulness." In the final sentence of her major book, *De Operatione Dei*, she said that the reason for her work was "for usefulness" (Fox, 1985).

Hildegard was a woman who, in spite of a patriarchal culture and a male-dominated church, strove to be heard. She struggled to offer her own wisdom and insights born of illumination from women of the past. Yet, now in our times, this woman author, healer, composer and mystic is honored and revered and her writings are being republished.

Nursing Nuns

By the 1300s hospitals and shelters for pilgrims and homes for the aged and poor multiplied throughout the continent. When leprosy developed in Europe, the order of St. Lazarus was organized specifically to nurse those afflicted with this disease. New orders of nursing nuns developed to care for other sick and poor. Health care during this era was nonscientific. It consisted of nurturing and caring, using herbs, potions, prayers, songs, and chants.

SCHOLASTICISM (1200 A.D. ONWARD)

As the centuries progressed, interest grew in a scientific approach to learning, and a method and system of thought referred to as scholasticism began. Since it continued to be a time of patriarchial domination, most of the recorded and revered work came from men. Scholars such as Albertus Magnus, Thomas Aquinas, and Duns Scotus Erigena began to systematize learning. They returned to the ancient roots of Greek philosophy and superimposed on those concepts the redeeming aspects of Christianity.

Between 1256 and 1272 Aquinas wrote a summary of these studies known as the *Summa* (summary). In this work he states that humans in their natural state, in this life, are an inseparable synthesis of spirit and body. Aquinas took the ancient knowledge of pagan and Arabic civilizations and showed that their wisdom was consistent with Christianity and that Christianity could add a new dimension to their reality. He opened the minds of his contemporaries to the philosophy of the ancients and of the Arabic world and reintroduced their science, mathematics, and medicine. It was this acceptance of the Arabic culture that brought us our modern numerical system (Arabic numerals), concepts of quantification, and eventually the emergence of empiricism, the scientific method, and modern technology.

As with all events through time there were ups and downs. In 1520 Henry VIII of England closed all the monasteries. As a result most of the unemployed monks went out and became physicians, and the nuns nurses, since healing was their skill. Thus the connecting link of the priest/priestess-healer was maintained, yet the link began to diminish as the ensuing year unfolded.

WISEWOMEN CRONES

During the age of faith there were several types of acknowledged healers: the priest-physicians, nursing-nuns, and the old wisewomen. It was the wise-women crones who cared for the vast majority of the day-to-day common ills. It was they who were the midwives tending pregnant women and delivering all the babies. It was they who passed the oral tradition of healing one to another. These women, steeped in ancient, ritualistic, and Druidic knowledge with the superimposed veneer of Christianity continued to incorporate nature and natural laws for healing purposes. Their use of herbs and potions and hands-on healing was invaluable during a time when most of humanity suffered with aches and pains of one kind or another.

Summary

The age of faith saw the further evolution of healers over a 1000-year period. Some were scholars, many were religious, but the vast majority were ordinary women guided by intuition and a sense of caring who answered a higher calling and developed the stamina and skills to care for the ill and infirm to the best of their abilities. Many of these people were precursers to those we can call nurse-healers today. The nurse healer of today derives strength from faith and a sense of vocation.

Healer Reflections

How would I feel as a nobleman or noblewoman as I decided to give up a royal life to dedicate myself to the care of others?

Have I ever received visions or illuminations like Hildegard of Bingen? If so, what have I done with them?

Can I imagine myself as a wise woman crone?

How it would feel to bring my intuitive knowledge and skills from the tenth into the twentith century?

REFERENCES

Donahue, M. P. *Nursing the finest art: An illustrated history.* St. Louis: C.V. Mosby, 1985.

Fox, M. *Illumination of Hildegard of Bingen.* Santa Fe, N. Mex.: Bear, 1985.

Reason and Science:
The Renaissance

*My nature is subdued to what it works in, so pity me then,
and wish I were renewed.*

William Shakespeare (1564–1616)

Empowering Yourself

Note the contrast in backgrounds from which healers arise. Some emerge from peasant stock while others come from the nobility.

Identify the period and the personal theory responsible for the dualistic mind and spirit split that affected healing then and is still operant in contemporary times.

Consider what factors influenced the decline of the role of the church in healing.

Learn about the nurse who was responsible for revolution-izing health care delivery in hospitals.

Become aware of the wide range of healing styles during this period of evolution.

HEALTH CARE PRACTICES

Toward the close of the age of faith and the beginning of the Renaissance there still continued to be an enormous amount of faulty knowledge and superstition regarding healing practice. The majority of these beliefs had been passed down from the ancient world and from tribal ancestors.

In the fourteenth and fifteenth centuries astrology and alchemy were still accepted practices. Physicians consulted the horoscope of their patients, as well as medical texts, to determine diagnosis and treatment. Astrological signs were used to determine when to take medicines or when to bleed the patient since bodily functions were supposedly controlled by the planets. Pharmacological treatment included use of exotics such as horn of the unicorn, powdered mummy, or crocodile dung. Leeches for bloodletting were an important part of therapy as the Renaissance began.

Epidemics continued to ravage Europe from the sixteenth to the nineteenth centuries. Outbreaks of typhus and bubonic plague reduced the population to only a fraction of its previous size. Approximately one third of the population of London died in the plagues that swept England in 1603 and 1625. Cholera epidemics occurred frequently, often wiping out huge populations in the slum areas of cities. Syphilis became so widespread that it too was considered one of the great plagues. As it became known that contracting the disease was related to sexual relations, social norms began to change rapidly.

THE FATE OF THE WISE WOMEN

During this era when men dominated the intellectual and political arena, it was the old wise women, the precursers of nurse healers, who used the intuitive, nonrational aspects of the mind for a different kind of healing. It was they who provided help for the masses and yet it was they who suffered banishment both by the church and the government. As they stood their ground against incriminating decrees, they risked heavy fines, excommunication, public whippings, and exile.

In an atmosphere of rapid change incited by a controversy over who should and should not minister to the sick, thousands of women were persecuted. While on the one hand Europe was beginning a renaissance of art and culture, on the other hand, it was the beginning of one of the saddest events in the history of healing and of women: the great witch hunt. In addition to other heinous acts, the wise women, now termed witches, were accused of having the magical power to affect health, both in their ability to heal, as well as to cause illness and death (Achterberg, 1985).

The church, which was very powerful and supported by the civil authorities, felt that all healing should be accomplished through their ministry. Healing without church supervision was felt to be under the influence of evil processes and evil spirits. There was a saying that "where God was not acknowledged, there was the presence of evil." The church was aware, however, of the power of incantations and talismans and therefore developed sacraments of the sick and the use of relics rather than talismans. Independent women who felt the power of the universe operating directly through them rather than through the mediation of the church came into obvious conflict with the establishment.

THE RENAISSANCE (1400 A.D. ONWARD)

The Renaissance began in Europe about 1400. It was a period of vigorous rebirth marked by the commitment of the educated classes to return to the classical cultures of ancient Greece and Rome. One of the primary outcomes of this new mode of thinking was a steady decline of the power of the Catholic church and an intense growth of interest in worldly affairs. During this period people wanted to explore different aspects of the world without the incessant reference to God. As the ordinary person's relationship to God diminished, materialism and skepticism increased.

The Renaissance period awakened a tremendous interest in classical literature and the arts. The interest in the arts and sciences had a positive influence on medical advancement. However, the materialistic, secular approach gradually eroded the essence of spirit from the realm of healing.

THE SCIENTIFIC REVOLUTION (1600 A.D. ONWARD)

Many scholars date the eve of the scientific revolution with the writings of the seventeenth century philosopher René Descartes (1596–1650). Descartes began with the premise that the mind must be able to know the world and that to do so, one must first eliminate all previously held belief systems and thought patterns. He believed his new system, based on skepticism and methodical order, would allow thinkers to achieve clarity and truth. This line of thinking, however, brought him to a depressing conclusion: there was nothing of which one could be certain.

Descartes's world-changing theory was that human thinking is purely mechanical. It confronts the world as a separate object. The problem to be studied is broken down into its component parts and studied "atomistically." Problem solving and knowledge consisted of reducing the object of study into its smallest parts and then summing the results to reach conclusions. The object and the observer were two distinct entities; the entire process was mechanical.

THE EIGHTEENTH CENTURY

During the eighteenth century, mechanization increased. Instruments were invented for measurement and inspection of the physical body. Laennec developed the stethoscope after listening to heart sounds through a tube of rolled-up paper tied with a string.

Psychiatry developed as a separate branch of medicine in the latter part of the eighteenth century. During the sixteenth and seventeenth centuries, it was believed that the mentally ill were possessed by demons. They were treated inhumanely, often cast out or locked up in cells.

As religion declined, so did the availability of religious hospitals. In Catholic countries such as Italy and Spain, there was not such a dele-terious result; however, in other areas of Europe, many small hospitals closed, leaving only the secular city hospitals. These municipal and state institutions were more like prisons than the old cloister hospitals of the Middle Ages with their beautiful gardens, roomy halls, and springs of water. By contrast, the secular hospitals of the seventeenth and eighteenth centuries were bare, undecorated, with small dark rooms and little ventilation or fresh air. There were dismal wards where fifty to a hundred patients were crowded together and cared for by nurses and assistants who had no formal training and were more often than not derelicts, drunks, and illiterates off the street who traded their services for room and board. This was in sharp contrast to the previous charitable institutions supported and run by those whose spiritual faith and healing intention guided their service.

THE NINETEENTH CENTURY

When hospital conditions were at their worst and the level of caregiving at its all-time low, a birth occurred that would affect the entire course of the future of healing.

Florence Nightingale, named after her city of birth, was born in Florence, Italy, on May 13, 1820. Her wealthy and influential English parents provided her with an excellent education. She and her sister were tutored by governesses, and by her early teens she had mastered the fundamentals of Latin, Greek, history, mathematics, and philosophy. She was shy and sensitive, unlike her more socially oriented sister, and liked to observe and write about the various places she visited on travels with her parents.

From an early age Florence expressed a desire to enter nursing, but her parents were convinced that it was a profession suited only for women of low social status with no education. They knew of the conditions in the hospitals and the type of women who worked there. Florence, however, true to her calling, felt that she had what it took to correct the evils so prevalent in nursing and, despite the objections of her parents, sought to learn all she could about the field. Her parents were dismayed that she rejected offers of marriage and the opportunity to assume her inherited place in society.

In 1851 at the age of 31 she resolved to finally do as she thought best and traveled to Kaiserwerth, Germany, where she stayed for 3 months of nurses' training. Her parents, who still objected, consented to the trip as long as where she had gone and why remained a secret among their own circle of friends. She returned to England via Paris where she toured hospitals and religious institutions and observed surgeons at work. Once back in England, her secret became public when she assumed the position of superintendent of the Establishment for Gentlewomen During Illness, a charity hospital for governesses run by titled ladies. Discontented with the board of directors, who had little knowledge of good hospital care, she left the position after a short period. As she was negotiating for a new position, the Crimean War broke out and an unexpected opportunity arose. Through her friends and acquaintances in high governmental positions she secured an appointment as superintendent of the Female Nursing Establishment of the English Hospitals in Turkey. In October 1854 Florence and thirty-eight self-proclaimed nurses of various experience departed for Scutari, a suburb of Constantinople in

Asia Minor. It was here at Scutari that Miss Nightingale made history.

The Barrack Hospital at Scutari was designed to accommodate 1700 patients, but between 3000 and 4000 suffering, wounded, and disabled soldiers were tightly packed into this hospital when Florence and her team arrived. There were 4 miles of beds situated 18 inches apart. The mattresses on the beds, the unwashed floor, and even parts of the wall were soaked with liquid excrement from the unchecked dysentery and cholera that so many of the inflicted developed. Lice, maggots, rats, and roaches crawled everywhere. It was a terrible mass of suffering humanity enmeshed in filth and disease that greeted the arriving group of thirty-nine nurses.

Initially, the resident physicians were not willing to allow Florence to begin the massive cleanup effort she proposed, but when they saw that she would withhold all service unless she was given complete control, they finally relented and let her begin. Within 10 days of arrival, she had set up a kitchen and converted a rented house into a laundry. All of the nurses scrubbed and cleaned, replaced filthy linen with clean, and cooked and served nutritious meals to the soldiers. In addition- they used their nursing skills to dress oozing and purulent wounds, fight fevers, and treat illnesses. Florence was determined to improve the sanitary conditions of the environment by attention to details, and she accomplished her objectives by separating different diseases into different sections, moving beds, opening windows, and airing the space. Once she had established order within the physical environment, she began a program of social welfare. Her staff assisted with letter writing and other comfort measures of the ill and dying.

During this time she also monitered her staff for their behavior. It was her intention that her nurses be moral and attentive only to their work. Some say she was disliked by a large percentage of her staff, yet she quickly developed the reputation for a thoroughness of care that saved lives and for accurate record keeping that showed how and why the care made a difference.

When she first arrived at the Barrack Hospital, the mortality rate was 60%; when she left it was only 1%. She was the first nurse who, through attention to detail demonstrated by record keeping, intention to heal, and perseverance of will, proved that quality nursing care made the difference between life and death.

On her return to England in 1856 she retired from frontline care and devoted herself to the pursuit of two goals. She spent the remainder of her life reforming the sanitary practices of the Army and establishing formal training schools for nurses. She returned to her parent's home and from the chaise lounge in her room received visitors of state, wrote two books, and in fact changed the course of the evolution of health care. Her most famous book was *Notes on Nursing* (1859), which, still enjoyed by students today, was the basis for formal nursing education that began as the result of her efforts.

HEALING WATERS

As we review history, we note the continuing correlation between physical sites and the occurrence of documented healings. In prerecorded history we saw that healing ceremonies took place with and around water. This practice continued even until recent times as healing centers such as Lourdes were erected around thermal springs, sea coasts, rivers, and lakes. The element of water is used to this day in rites of purification ceremonies. For example, simple, routine bathing techniques are still used in the most sophisticated healing centers of the modern world.

Summary

Five hundred years of evolution have been condensed into a brief summary within the confines of this chapter. These 500 years were filled with drama, passion, pestilence, plague, and disease. There were incredible strides forward and heavy losses in terms of the divorce of spirit from Western mainstream healing practice.

Healer Reflections

How could I defend myself if my nursing techniques were equated with practicing witchcraft?

If I had the opportunity, as did Florence Nightingale, to stand up for what I believed, would I?

Do I know of or am working on some scientific process that, if applied, could better the quality of life for others?

Can I think of ways to reinstill art into nursing?

REFERENCES

Achterberg, J. *Imagery in healing.* Boston: New Science Library, 1985.

Kalish, P. A. & Kalisch, B. J. *The advance of American nursing.* Boston: Little, Brown, 1978.

Minkowski, W. Women healers of the middle ages: Selected aspects of their history. *American Journal of Public Health,* 1992, *82* (2), 288–295.

Shealy, M. C. Florence Nightingale 1820–1910, An evolutionary mind in the context of holism. *Journal of Holistic Nursing*, 1985, *3* (1), 4–6.

The Advent of Holism: Contemporary Healers

A healer is no passive observer. She or he sees people whose bodies are disintegrating, whose lives have lost their safety. . . . It is the impulse to commonplace courage and everyday heroism that the healer formalizes into a life's work.

John Poppy

Empowering Yourself

Note why it was difficult for healers to emerge from the early years of American culture.

Identify the decade that the pendulum had swung the limit with illness being perceived as a strictly pathophysiological event.

Identify some of the pioneers of the twentieth century who awakened the concept of whole-body healing.

THE NEW WORLD VIEW

By the nineteenth century the Cartesian approach of dividing mind into one compartment and body and spirit into others was well integrated into the healing arts of the Western world. Professionals, who had developed into the class of recognized and acknowledged healers, followed scientific curricula and worked diligently to serve the sick using their best scientific approaches. The religious communities continued to educate many nurses and maintained the heritage of embodying spiritual practices in their care of patients.

In the early years of American history both professional and lay healers suffered serious setbacks. The complexities of the evolution from an agrarian to an industrialized society, coupled with the cities' burgeoning immigrant population, left little time for whole-health concerns. Early American health care workers were battling with sanitation, basic hygiene, and immunization to combat the serious physical health problems. Again, with the exception of the religious hospitals, less and less time was available for inclusion of the mental and spiritual aspects of healing.

Increasing division between the professional healers' roles, increasing specialization within the divisions, and decreasing recognition of lay healers pushed the concept of whole-body healing farther and farther into the recess of the past. The more specialized and technical the delivery systems became, the less attention was alloted to the spiritual aspect. With the exception of the work of an isolated few, by the 1960s it appeared that the pendulum had swung the limit. Illness was perceived as a strictly pathophysiological event with the cure being completely allopathic, that is, based on a treatment of using remedies that produce effects opposite from those produced by the disease being treated.

It was during the early days of the new professional curricula that another decline and ultimate dissolution of feminine influence on the delivery of health care occurred. As the curricula grew in scientific content, so did the decrease in the feminine aspects of nurturance, intuition, and empathy. These qualities were seen as threats and impediments to the progression of the new scientific order.

REAWAKENING OF HOLISM

Throughout the decades it was the work of an isolated few who kept the concept of wholeness alive. The term holistic health was first introduced in South Africa in 1926. Prime Minister Jan Smuts, who had an intense interest in health, theorized that nature tends to bring things together to whole organisms and that the detemining factors in nature and evolution are wholes and not their constituent parts (Berman, 1981).

The awakening of the concept of holism to the health care community probably began in the 1940s with Dunbar (1945), a pioneer in psychosomatic medicine published studies relating personality type and stress to physical illness. Hans Selye (1956) followed with documentation about the psychophysiology of stress. He contended that when one does not cope adequately with stresses of life, diseases of adaptation, both mental or physical, will occur. Holmes and Raye (1967) followed by contributing what are currently classic studies that relate a point value of life stressors to the onset of illness and disease.

Nursing Theory

Martha Rogers (1970) set the precedent for holistic nursing theories with the introduction of her philosophy of the Science of Unitary Human Beings. Other theorists followed building and expanding on the theory of expanding consciousness and holistic integration. Parse (1981), Newman (1986), and Watson (1988) developed the themes of self-transcendence, open systems, space-time relativity, and evolution of consciousness. The significance of body, mind, spirit, and consciousness became an integral part of the art and science of nursing.

THE WELLNESS PARADIGM

In the early 1960s Halpert Dunn (1961) addressed the topic of wellness. His now classic definition of what he termed "high-level wellness" was "an integrated method of functioning which is oriented toward maximizing the potential of which the individual is capable within the environment where he is functioning." Dunn stressed that wellness was an ongoing process toward higher potential, not a static goal. High-level wellness was a feeling of being "alive to the tips of the fingers, with energy to burn, tingling with vitality." He postulated that health professionals tend to focus on disease rather than wellness or prevention because it is easier to fight against sickness than to fight for a condition of greater wellness.

An increase in the momentum, number, and scope of holistic practitioners began in the late 1970s. These practitioners, many of whom were nurses, began to weave in the thread of living a wellness life-style as a major factor in the health process. New techniques were tried and new ways explored. Major emphasis was on four major dimensions: nutrition, physical awareness, stress reduction, and self-responsibility. Out of this new practice, books and research emerged that helped influence the way Americans conceptualized health and healing.

THE HOLISTIC HEALTH MOVEMENT IN PROFESSIONAL ASSOCIATIONS

During the 1980s there was such a burgeoning interest in the concept of whole-body healing that some pioneering professionals and laity began to form associations and groups. In 1980 Charlotte McGuire founded the American Holistic Nurses' Association. This organization was the first to bring whole-person healing back into mainstream American nursing. The purpose of this association is to promote the education of nurses and the public in the concerns and practice of health of the whole person. Through the dedicated work of this organization, nurses have once again taken up the role of healer and seek to reunite the concepts of body, mind, and spirit in all aspects of nursing practice.

The new evolution of whole-body healing is based on whole-brain thinking. As we continue to evolve into wholeness, we base many of our new beliefs on empiricism but also take into account those ineffable, immeasurable, nonmaterial, and spiritual values that were the motivating factors of our predecessors in their search for truth. The world of empiricism has yielded valuable insight and should continue to be used, but our efforts must be blended with an understanding of the higher level of spirit. Our objective now is to learn from the past to help restore balance, for true science combines the philosophical sciences with the natural sciences. In this way we may return to our ancient roots in which all healing is based.

NURSING RESEARCH

Many nurse researchers are gathering data that contribute to the concept of the nurse as healer. Rew (1989) discusses dialoging with the transpersonal self as an exercise to enhance intuition and spiritual growth. Rees (1992) discovered that the use of guided imagery and relaxation assists new mothers in achieving maternal role attainment, while Heise (1993) describes the concept of the valuing process as it relates to structuring the meaning of individual health. These are but a few of many new research projects that utilize holistic theory to study and define new concepts.

Nurse researchers currently involved in a Delphi study have ascertained that the following guiding principles are a part of the contemporary nurse healers' practice (Freel & Estby, 1992). These principles are as follows:

1. There is a unity and interdependence within the mind, body, and spirit.

2. Health is a process that may include dis-ease.

3. One's attitudes and beliefs toward life (mental-emotional energy fields or consciousness) is a major etiological factor in health and disease.

4. One's health and disease are manifested in one's life-style, habits, and conscious awareness, as well as the body's physical being and energy.

5. The self is empowered with the ability to create or maintain health/disease.

6. Changes in health can occur through experiential learning. Experiential learning is defined as a change in behavior that occurs as a result of living through an activity, event, or situation.

7. Experiential learning is essential to changing one's life-style for high-level wellness.

8. Human beings are energy fields.

9. Healing involves a transformational change that encompasses the whole person; it requires the involvement of the spiritual, emotional, and intellectual domains, as well as the physical body.

10. Energy fields can become unbalanced as a response to stress in any one of the three domains of body, mind, and spirit.

11. The client-practitioner relationship is one of partnership—equal with differing responsibilities.

12. Any modality or health system that supports healing should be valued.

13. Each health system should be respected for the resources and the tools that it offers while being challenged to prove its credibility.

14. Each person is an open system with the environment without separating boundaries.

15. Energy fields are constantly interacting.

16. Health is the dynamic evolution toward balanced integration.

17. Health involves a sense of unity with the self and cosmos.

18. Wellness encompasses increasing openness (acceptance of diversity) and increasing harmony (coherent, high-frequency energy fields).

19. Health is influenced by the environment (interpenetrating external energy fields) and genetics (transgenerational energy fields).

20. Healing, when viewed holistically, is not predictable in terms of time frame, cause, or outcome.

21. The division of the whole person into three domains of body, mind, and spirit is an old-paradigm illusion.

22. Body, mind, and spirit share one consciousness.

23. The human spirit is the core of the person.

24. Spiritual health is necessary for physical, mental, and emotional well-being.

25. The Source is experienced or known through joy, beauty, love, light, peace, power, and life.

Summary

Throughout the 1980s there was a continual renaissance and blending of the healing techniques of antiquity (use of herbs, purification ceremonies, dream work, and so forth), the healing techniques of the Eastern world (meditation, acupuncture, and other meridian system therapies), and the scientific, empirical approach of the West. Individuals schooled in all approaches, with an appreciation of the lessons of history, have emerged from this cultural, temporal potpourri to teach and lead us as we travel the path to becoming nurse healers.

Because of the brevity of space, very few individuals have been cited as contemporary healers when in fact they abound everywhere. During the 1980s our cognition and intuition developed so rapidly that many individuals developed the qualities and attributes of healers. There has been an outpouring of written literature and oral presentations from hundreds of articulate spokespeople. Thousands of others have developed private clinical practices or work through other creative modes to express these reemerging healing qualities. It is the work of this book to further elucidate and articulate what these special qualities are so that we can imbibe them, thereby furthering the process of evolution for us all.

Healer Reflections

Do I feel empowered as I gain knowledge about healing from a cultural and historical perspective?

Do I understand the major role of nurses in the reawakening of holistic thought in contemporary practice?

Am I engaged in practice, education, or research that will contribute to the ongoing advance of nurse healing?

REFERENCES

Dunbar, F. *Psychomatic diagnosis.* New York: Paul B. Haeber, 1945.

Dunn, H. *High level wellness.* Arlington, Va: R.W. Beatty, 1961.

Freel, M. & Estby, S. Research Presentation, 12th Annual Conference, American Holistic Nurses' Association, Hot Springs, Ark., 1992.

Heise, J. L. The valuing process. *Journal of Holistic Nursing,* 1993, *11* (1), 56–63.

Holmes, T. H. Schedule of recent experience. Department of Psychiatry and Behavioral Sciences, University of Washington, Seattle, 1976.

Newman, M. *Health as expanding consciousness.* St. Louis: C.V. Mosby, 1986.

Parse, R. *Nursing science: Major paradigms, theories, and critiques.* Philadelphia: W.B. Saunders, 1987.

Rees, B. L. Using relaxation with guided imagery to assist primiparas in achieving maternal role attainment. *Journal of Holistic Nursing,* 1992, *10* (2), 167–182.

Rew, L. Intuition: Nursing knowledge and the spiritual dimensions of persons. *Holistic Nursing Practice,* 1989, *3* (3), 56–68.

Rogers, M. *The theoretical basis of nursing.* Philadelphia: F.A. Davis, 1970.

Selye, H. *The stress of life.* New York: McGraw-Hill, 1956.

Watson, J. *Nursing: Human science and human care.* New York: The National League for Nursing, 1988.

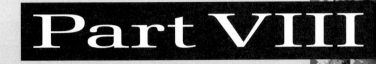

Part VIII

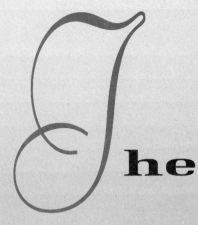

The
Creative
Practitioner

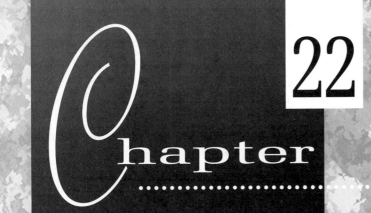

Chapter 22

The Creative Practitioner

The creative practitioner is a healer who recognizes the need for and develops the art of blending the components of linear and intuitive, theory and practice, and art and science into whole-brain thinking. This practitioner has learned that the healing of others is based on an inherent wholeness of the self—physically, mentally, and spiritually. The path to wholeness is a process in itself, and as a process it is continually unfolding as individual consciousness expands to encompass increased vision of the possible.

LINEAR AND INTUITIVE THOUGHT PATTERNS

Whole-brain thinking is comprised of blending the linear and intuitive thought processes. The human brain is composed of two primary cognitive hemispheres, the so-called right brain and left brain. Although both sides are equal in weight and dimension, Western medicine labels the left hemisphere the dominant hemisphere because the left side of our brain controls and regulates the valued, linear actions of an ordered, productive life. Linear refers to the reasoning, logical, verbal, mathematical, calculative aspect of thinking. The intuitive processes, on the other hand, are regulated by the right hemisphere. Intuitive function has to do with creativity, artistry, poetry, and the knowing-without-knowing-why aspects of our cognition and behavior. Both aspects are important and both can be developed. Specific skills can be practiced to develop either right or left hemisphere functions. When they are both developed and integrated, one becomes a whole-brain thinker. It is the goal of holistic practitioners to blend the two equally important dimensions and operate from this base of whole-brain thinking.

HEALING FROM A BASE OF WHOLENESS

Throughout this text we have witnessed accounts of healing from a variety of perspectives. Despite the differences in approach and/or technique, there are common threads that connect all healers. The commonality that unites them is the universal intent for healing or assisting another person to an outcome consistent with a greater good, and the realization of the interconnectedness of all things. The trait of intent to heal includes cure of illness, as well as acceptance of disease and transition to the dimension beyond the physical form. Interconnectedness includes matter, as well as mind and spirit. Most healers pattern by the classical archetypes; a few, however, follow their own different drummer and will therefore evolve new archetypes as we continue to evolve as a species.

PERSONAL CHARACTERISTICS OF HEALERS

We have witnessed a variety of healers in a number of situations throughout this text. It is important to note that these healers are not idealized gods and goddesses with perfect figures and no personal problems. Although an archetype or multiple archetypes may exist within an individual, the person is still human and, as a human, still struggles with temporal problems and physical ills and imbalances.

There are all kinds of healers. You may meet a broken-nosed, thick-spectacled, pot-bellied, balding individual that superficially you might be inclined to dismiss based on personal appearance. Yet if you observe closely enough over a period, you may be amazed by that person's prowess. Others may seem absent-minded, forgetful, and disorganized and then suddenly surprise you with healing ability. There are even narcissistic, self-centered people who, given particular settings with particular focus away from self, actually provide significant healing results. The point is that we must not be too quick to judge another's healing abilities. Healers come in all shapes and sizes. Although most healers portray archetypes, not many come in godlike or goddesslike physical packages. We cannot know another's capacities merely by cursory observation.

To become a healer we must focus on developing certain attitudes and behaviors in ourselves. Do we possess the attitudes of joy, caring, and purpose? Do we live with authenticity, being fully present as we empathetically listen and perform service with attention to detail? As we heal, we become increasingly cognizant of blending the linear and intuitive domains as we holistically express our intent through the hands, from the heart, and with the spirit. Those who master these attitudes and behaviors are on the path to becoming a healer.

HEALING IN THE NEW MILLENNIUM

It is paradoxical, but at this time in our evolution we, as a society, are simultaneously functioning in three distinct health delivery paradigms. Dossey (1989) describes three eras of medicine operant in the West. Era I is technological and is based on the pathophysiological system of cause and effect. In many institutional settings this is the mode of current conceptualization and concurrent medical practice. It is true that Era I has led to miraculous breakthroughs in diagnosis and treatment, but at a cost. For one thing it is wildly expensive. In addition it has made little advance against catastrophic illness while at the same time it has become increasingly impersonal and intrusive. Some, like Dossey, forecast that the health care delivery system, as we know it in Era I, is at the end of its time.

Era II medicine, operant in some contemporary settings, utilizes the mind-body connection and takes into account psychological principles and the effect of emotions on psychophysiology and pathophysiology. Bodywork, biofeedback laboratories, and settings that utilize music, aesthetics, and laughter are all part of the emerging Era II domain. Dossey predicts Era III medicine to be the norm in the new millennium. Era III is based on the metaphysical concept of the development of changes in consciousness occurring prior to changes in matter and energy.

We are in the midst of paradigm shifts. Eras I, II, and III are in flux and the best of all three will likely result in Era IV. We are at the threshold of awakening as stewards of all our resources, both inner and outer. We are at the place where science, medicine, and spirituality will be embraced by those with healing attitudes to create new possibilities for all people. As this shift advances, emphasis for both the individual and society will be on achieving maximum wellness.

Many of the oncoming changes will evolve from societal changes. These include demographic, economic, science, and technology. There will be, for example, increasing numbers of elderly and intensifying diversity from continuing immigration. The economy and science will support new health care options. Technology will continue to advance as we move into the twenty-first century. To realize the speed with which technology has developed, consider that as recently as 1970 computer chips did not even exist. Today, there are more of these chips than people on the earth.

As we advance, society will see itself in the image of a complex organism and, as such, will begin to design health care communities as living organic wholes. We can expect the emergence of renewal centers dedicated to healing; these centers will be reminiscent of the Greek Askepilons. Today 80% to 90% of all those who seek medical attention do not have organic disease. They do have symptoms and do seek therapy, but there is no pathology. There are already some sites where these people can go for nontraditional treatment and others are on the threshold of developing the kinds of healing centers that would benefit them. These are centers that would address the problem of symptoms without pathology or disease and the prevention of disease emergence.

Nursing Centers

Many healers are in the process of conceptualizing the kind of therapy centers needed. Nursing centers are poised to become primary sites for future health care delivery. Nursing centers that become healing centers and the nurse healers who staff them will focus on self-responsibility and viewing illness and symptoms as opportunities for growth. Future health centers will contain all the finest elements of antiquity but will house and utilize the most modern technology. There will be, for example, flotation tanks, quadraphonic-sound relaxation units, light and color therapy, and biofeedback devices, just to name a few. These units will be planned in ecological settings and utilize both professional and lay people.

Healing will evolve from the unifocused sterile, technological mode of the modern hospital into high-tech, high-touch care with a multidimensional focus on body, mind and spirit. There will be new modes of therapy that include a variety of new practices. Health care delivery will include such things as music, imagery, energy movement, humor, food, and friendship. In the new millennium a new definition of healing will emerge that includes caring alongside curing.

The Nurse Healer

As we widen our perception, we recognize that healers are all around us. They may be in out-patient departments, intensive care units, home health, school nursing, or in research or education. Any nurse, given the right attitudes and behaviors can become a nurse healer. One who works for integration of the totality of humankind in body, mind, and spirit in any health care setting attempts healing. Those who become nurse healers refine their natural abilities and are capable of producing or catalyzing that integration.

Nurses have come a long way in a few short decades. In the past our attention focused on physical, mental, and emotional healing. Now we talk of healing your life, healing the environment, and healing the planet. Our vision of healing and what it means to lead a healing life has broadened dramatically. Abraham Maslow (1971) stated that the work of nurses was probably one of the finest examples of peak experiences in daily living. Those who have had peak experiences have gone beyond or transcended the self-actualization level on his classical, theoretical, pyramid level of motivation. The orginal levels of motivation, well known to nurses, included in order: physiological needs, safety needs, belonging, self-esteem, and self-actualization. The following are characteristics of self-actualized people for whom peak experiences are central:

- Serene, calm experiences of transcendence are central in their lives.
- They speak the language of Being.
- They perceive the unity of life and see both the sacred and practical in everyday life.
- They are able to recognize one another.
- They are inspiring.
- They are innovators.
- They are sensitive to the problems in the world.
- They see the sacredness of every person and every living thing.
- They see the mystery in life.
- They have an understanding of evil in the world.
- They view themselves as instruments of the transpersonal.
- They are more accepting of people who are different.
- They are more responsive to beauty.
- They are more holistic, synergistic, and more spiritual.

Nurse scientists have since built on Maslow's classical work. Sarter (1988) in analyzing contemporary nursing theories points out that the evolution of human consciousness leads to self-transcendence and unity with all. Barnum (1989) studied the experiences of expanded consciousness of 118 nursing leaders. She found that 41% of the participants reported one or more experiences of expanded consciousness. This and other recent studies indicate that nurses are moving into the forefront of consciousness and the arena of a transcendent practice. Many nurses already direct their practice from this vantage point. Thousands of others are poised on the threshold waiting to follow the lead and move into a new perception of a new dimension of healing in the new millennium.

Healing attitudes and behaviors, as well as interconnectedness and wholeness, are being applied to the earth as an living organism. The concept of healing as making whole is rapidly emerging as a force in world politics. Visionary nurse healers are leading the way in helping to redefine what it means to heal and to make whole.

REFERENCES

Barnum, B. J. Expanded consciousness: Nurses' experiences. *Nursing Outlook,* 1989, *37* (6), 260–266.

Dossey, L. *Recovering the soul.* New York: Bantam Books, 1989.

Maslow, A. *The farther reaches of human nature.* New York: Viking Press, 1971.

Sarter, M. Philosophical sources of nursing theory. *Nursing Science Quarterly, 1988, 1* (2), 52–59.

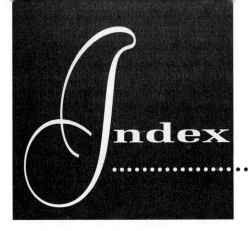

Index